THE GASTRIC SLEEVE BARIATRIC COOKBOOK For BEGINNERS

Easy Meal plans,Effortless and Delicious Recipes to Enjoy Favourite Foods Before and After Weight-Loss Surgery

INTRODUCTION

WHAT IS BARIATRIC SURGERY?

Bariatric surgery is an operation that by making improvements to your digestive system, helps you lose weight. Some forms of bariatric surgery make the stomach smaller, allowing you to eat and drink all at once, helping you feel full faster. The small intestine, the portion of the body that consumes calories and nutrients from foods and liquids, is often modified by other bariatric surgeries.

If you have extreme obesity and have not been able to lose weight or keep from gaining back any weight you lost using other therapies such as lifestyle therapy or drugs, bariatric surgery may be an option. Bariatric surgery can also an option if you have severe obesity-related health issues, such as type 2 diabetes or sleep apnea. Many medical conditions linked to obesity, especially type 2 diabetes, can be improved by bariatric surgery.

DOES BARIATRIC SURGERY ALWAYS WORK?

Studies show that, depending on the type of operation they have many individuals who have bariatric surgery lose an average of around 15 to 30 percent of their starting weight. No system, however is sure to produce and sustain weight loss, including surgery. Some individuals with bariatric surgery do not lose as much as they thought they would. Some individuals recover a portion of the weight they lost over time. There may be differences in the amount of weight people recover. Factors affecting weight recovery may include the level of obesity of an individual and the type of surgery he or she has had.

Bariatric surgery does not substitute healthier habits, but it does make it easier for you to eat and be more physically active with less calories. Before and after the surgery, choosing healthier foods and drinks will help you lose more weight and hold it off in the long term. Regular after-surgery physical exercise also helps to keep the weight off. You must commit to a lifetime of healthy lifestyle practices and follow the recommendations of your healthcare providers to improve your health.

BARIATRIC COOKBOOK RECIPES

1.CHEESY CHICKEN AND BROCCOLI CASSEROLE

Prep:15 mins

Cook:35 mins

Total:50 mins

Ingredients

- 1 tsp unsalted butter
- Two skinless, boneless chicken breasts, cubed
- 3 cups of finely chopped broccoli
- 10.5 ounce condensed cream of chicken soup
- 1 cup of shredded Cheddar cheese
- 1 cup of shredded Parmesan cheese, divided
- ½ cup of shredded mozzarella cheese
- ½ cup of sour cream
- ground black pepper, as need

Directions

1. Heat the oven to 350 degrees F. Butter a 9x13-inch dish on the bottom and sides.
2. Get it to a boil with a pot of water. Add the chicken and continue to boil for 5 to 10 minutes, until it is no longer pink.
3. Meanwhile, in a big bowl, add broccoli, chicken soup cream, Cheddar cheese, 1/2 cup Parmesan cheese, mozzarella, sour cream, and pepper. Mix thoroughly.
4. Drain the chicken and add a mixture of broccoli. Mix thoroughly. Pour into the baking dish prepared and spread evenly.

5. Bake for 20 minutes in the preheated oven. Add the remaining Parmesan cheese and continue to bake for 3 to 5 minutes until the cheese is melted.

Cook's Notes:

- Instead of fresh, if desired, you can use thawed, frozen broccoli.
- After baking for 20 minutes, you can sprinkle whatever cheese you want on top.

Nutrition Info
Per Serving :

protein 18.3g; 265 calories, carbohydrates 9.1g; fat 17.4g ; cholesterol 55.8mg ; sodium 832.4mg

2. FAT-FREE REFRIED BEANS

Prep:10 mins

Cook:15 mins

Total:25 mins

Ingredients

- 2 cups of canned black beans, divided
- ½ cup of water
- 2 cloves minced garlic
- 1 tsp pepper
- 1 tsp salt
- 1 tsp liquid smoke flavouring
- ¾ cup of diced onion

Directions

1. Mash 2/3 of a cup of beans into a smooth paste in a small bowl.
2. Combine the remaining beans with the water in a medium saucepan over medium heat. Stir in garlic, pepper, salt, and liquid smoke when thoroughly heated.
3. Stir in the whole beans with the bean paste and combine well. Stir in the onion and cook for about 10 minutes or until lightly cooked.

Nutrition Info

Per Serving:

protein 7.7g,134 calories, sodium 1044.4mg, carbohydrates 23.3g, fat 1.5g, cholesterol 0mg

3. GREEK SPINACH BAKE

Total Time

Prep: 10 min. Bake: 1 hour

Ingredients

- 2 cups of cottage cheese
- 10 ounces frozen, thawed, and squeezed dry chopped spinach
- 8 ounces crumbled feta cheese
- 6 tbsp all-purpose flour
- 1/2 tsp pepper
- 1/4 tsp salt
- Four large lightly beaten eggs

Directions

1. Combine the cottage cheese, the spinach, and the feta cheese in a wide bowl: incorporate the flour, pepper, and salt. Add the eggs and combine well.
2. Spoon into a 9-in, greased one—a square dish for baking. Bake until a thermometer reads 160 degrees F, about 1 hour, uncovered, at 350 degrees F.

Nutrition Info

1 each: 262 calories, 178mg cholesterol,13g fat, 838mg sodium, 14g carbohydrate, 21g protein.

4. KETO CHICKEN CRUST PIZZA

Prep:10 mins

Cook:35 mins

Total:45 mins

Ingredients

- 1 pound ground chicken
- ½ cup of shredded mozzarella cheese
- ¼ cup of freshly grated Parmesan cheese
- 3 cloves minced garlic
- 1 tsp Italian seasoning
- ½ tsp salt
- ¼ tsp pepper
- 1 tbsp chopped fresh basil

Directions

1. Heat the oven to 400 degrees F.Line a parchment paper baker.
2. In a big bowl, mix chicken, mozzarella cheese, Parmesan cheese, garlic, Italian seasoning, salt, and pepper. Fold in basil chopped.
3. Place the chicken mix between two parchment paper pieces. Spread the mixture from 1/4-1/2-inch thick into a circle or rectangle. Remove top paper parchment.
4. Bake in a preheated oven for 35 to 45 minutes, until the edges start to brown. Top your favourite tapestries.

Nutrition Info

Per Serving:

409 calories, fat 14.6g, Protein 62g, carbohydrates 4.1g, cholesterol 165.2mg, sodium 1030.3mg.

5. TACO CASSEROLE

Prep Time: 15 minutes

Cook Time: 30 minutes

Total Time: 45 minutes

Ingredients

- 2 tsp olive oil
- 1 pound ground beef
- 1/2 cup of onion finely diced
- 1 packet taco casserole
- 14.5 ounce can diced tomatoes do not drain
- 1 1/4 cups of tortilla chips crushed
- 16 ounce can refried beans
- 1 1/4 cups of cheddar cheese shredded
- Toppings such as shredded lettuce, diced tomato, and sliced olives
- cooking spray

INSTRUCTIONS

1. Heat the oven to 350 degrees F. Cover with cooking spray a 9-inch square pan or 2-quart baking dish.
2. Heat olive oil over medium heat in a big pot. Add ground beef and cook for 5-6 minutes, and spatula the meat.
3. Add onion and cook 3-4 minutes or until the onion is translucent.
4. Stir the taco seasoning and the tomatoes diced. Simmer three to four minutes. Simmer.
5. Place a tortilla layer on the bottom of the prepared pan. Spread a sheet of cooled beans on top.
6. Place the mix of beef on the beans and add the cheese.

7. Bake for 20 minutes, or melted cheese.
8. If you want to add toppings, then serve.

NUTRITION INFO

Calories: 435kcal, Carbohydrates: 31g, Protein: 26g, Fat: 20g , Saturated Fat: 8g, Cholesterol: 73mg, Iron: 4.1mg Sodium: 709mg, Potassium: 465mg, Fiber: 6g, Sugar: 5g, Vitamin A: 925IU, Vitamin C: 10mg, Calcium: 270mg

6. CRAB RANGOON WONTON ROLLS

prep time: 10 MINUTES

cook time: 20 MINUTES

total time: 30 MINUTES

INGREDIENTS

- 12 wonton wrappers
- 12 ounces softened cream cheese
- ¼ cup of sour cream
- 4 ounces imitation crab, substitute 1 can drain lump crab
- 2 green thinly sliced onions
- ¼ tsp. Worcestershire sauce
- ¼ tsp. soy sauce

INSTRUCTIONS

1. Heat the oven to 350 degrees F.
2. Spray the cooking spray muffin pan.
3. Place one wrapper in each cup of a muffin; bake before the edges begin to brown for 10 minutes.
4. Remove slightly from the oven and cool.
5. Mix cream cheese, sour cream, 1 green onion, Worcestershire, and soy sauce in a medium bowl. Stir well. Stir well.
6. In a small food processor, place crab and process until finely chopped. Mix the chopped crab in the mixture of cream cheese.
7. Fill the spoon in the shells of baked wonton; Bake for another 8-12 minutes.
8. Cover with green onions in slices. Serve with chilli sweet and savoury or sweet as needed.

NOTES

- Using 8 oz for a more concentrated crab taste. Cheese cream and 8 oz. Crab imitation and keep other measurements similar.

NUTRITION INFO:

Amount Per Serving:

CALORIES: 150, FIBER: 0g, TOTAL FAT: 11g, CARBOHYDRATES: 8g, SATURATED FAT: 6g, TRANS FAT: 0g, UNSATURATED FAT: 3g, CHOLESTEROL: 44mg, SODIUM: 233mg, SUGAR: 2g, PROTEIN: 5g

7. BROCCOLI AND RICOTTA PANCAKES

Total: 25 min

Active: 25 min

Ingredients

- 2 cups of pureed broccoli
- 1 1/2 cups of ricotta cheese
- 1 1/2 cups of all-purpose flour
- 1 tbsp olive oil
- 1 tsp baking powder
- 2 large beaten eggs
- Kosher salt
- 3 tbsp salted butter

Directions

1. Heat the oven to 200 degrees F.
2. In a large mixing bowl, combine broccoli, ricotta, meal, olive oil, baking powder, egg, and salt with a wooden spoon.
3. Working in batches, melt some butter over medium heat in a cast-iron or nonstick pan. Ladle dollops in the batter's pan to accommodate as many as you can at one time without them sticking together. Cook 2 to 3 minutes per hand, depending on your pan, and heat until browned on each side. Make the cooked ones as you work and keep them warm in the oven as needed. Continue with the batter and butter left. With a little more butter, we serve the pancakes hot.

Cook's Note

- The broccoli purée is just broccoli with a little water purified by steam. We still try to cook more broccoli to consume more vegetables and know that it will suit somewhere.

8. LOW CARB BIG MAC BITES

prep time: 20 MINS

cook time: 15 MINS

total time: 35 MINS

INGREDIENTS

- 1.5 pounds Ground beef
- ¼ cup of finely diced Onion
- 1 tsp Salt
- 4 slices American Cheese
- 16 slices Dill Pickle
- Lettuce

SECRET SAUCE

- 1/2 cup of Mayonnaise
- 4 tbsp Dill pickle relish
- Yellow mustard (2 tbsp)
- White wine vinegar (1 tsp)
- Paprika (1 tsp)
- 1 tsp Onion powder
- 1 tsp Garlic powder

INSTRUCTIONS

1. Heat the oven to 400 degrees F.
2. Combine ground beef, onions, and salt in a large bowl. Mix until fully mixed. Mix.
3. Roll the beef into 1.5 balls of an ounce. Press each to flatten it slightly to make a mini burger patty and place it onto a baker's sheet.
4. Bake for 15 minutes or until cooked, at 400 degrees F.
5. While cooking burgers, add all the secret sauce ingredients in a bowl and mix.
6. Turn off the oven when the burgers are baked and remove them—Pat same grateful abundance.
7. Cut each slice of cheese into four squares and place a piece on every mini patty. Return to the cooling oven and let the cheese melt.
8. Place some squares of lettuce and a bowl on top of each meatball and run through it with a skewer.
9. Serve the secret sauce and have fun!

NUTRITION INFO

serving: 1skewer, calories: 182kcal, carbohydrates: 1g, protein: 10g, fat: 12g, saturated fat: 4g, polyunsaturated fat: 3g, monounsaturated fat: 2g, sodium: 414mg, cholesterol: 36mg, potassium: 26mg, vitamin a: 23iu, vitamin c: 1mg, calcium: 75mg, iron: 6mg

9. HEALTHY CHOCOLATE HUMMUS

Prep Time: 10 minutes

Total Time: 10 minutes

Ingredients

- 2 cup of chickpeas
- 4 tbsp unsweetened cocoa powder
- 2 tbsp all-natural peanut butter
- 1/4 cup of pure maple syrup
- 1 tsp vanilla extract

Instructions

1. Add all ingredients to a broad food processor cup and purée smoothly.
2. Serve with fresh fruit, crackers, or chips of pita.

Nutrition

Calories: 147kcal, Sodium: 226mg, Carbohydrates: 23g, Protein: 6g, Fat: 5g, Saturated Fat: 1g, Fiber: 5g, Sugar: 9g

10. PROTEIN BREAKFAST COOKIES

prep time: 20 minutes

total time: 20 minutes

INGREDIENTS

- 1/2 cup of almond butter
- 1/2 cup of pure maple syrup
- 2/3 cup + 1 tbsp Kodiak Cakes Power Cakes Buttermilk Mix
- 1 scoop vanilla protein powder
- 1/2 tsp pure vanilla extract
- 1 tbsp ground cinnamon
- 1/8 tsp fine sea salt

Optional white chocolate drizzle

- 1/4 cup of white chocolate chips
- 1/2 tsp coconut oil
- 1/16 tsp ground cinnamon

INSTRUCTIONS

1. *Cookies*: Combine in a large bowl 1/2 cup of almond butter, 1/2 cup of pure maple syrup, 2/3 cups + 1 tbsp of Kodiak mix, 1 scooping protein powder, 1/2 tsp extract of vanilla, 1 tbsp of cinnamon ground, and 1/8 tsp of fine sea salt. Combine well with a hand blender or a wooden spoon.
2. *SCOOP*: To measure dough, use a 1-inch cookie scoop. You should have about 40 balls. You can pause and enjoy them as protein bites or continue to make cookies.

3. **FROM**: Force the balls to form a small cookie. Put on a paper-lined parchment tray.
4. **OPTIONAL WHITE CHOCOLATE DRIZZL**E: Mix 1/4 cup white chocolate chips with 1/2 tsp of coconut oil in a small bowl (measure when melted). Microwave up to melted and smooth in 15 seconds. Stir in 1/16 tsp cinnamon ground. Transfer to a small bag and cut off the end of the corner with a small tip. Pip a swirl overall cookies.
5. **STORAGE**: Facilitate the hardening of white chocolate at room temperature. Then tightly cover cookies and store them in the refrigerator or freezer. I place them in a small airtight bag in the freezer and take a bag to the fridge to have fun.

NUTRITION INFO

Serving:

Calories:41kcal, Fiber:0.4g, Carbohydrates:5.2g, Protein:1.3g , Fat:1.8g, Sodium:30.8mg, Cholesterol:0.1mg, Sugar:2.9g

11. STEAK FAJITA BELL PEPPER BOATS

PREP TIME: 1 hr 10 mins

COOK TIME: 15 mins

TOTAL TIME: 1 hr 25 mins

INGREDIENTS

- 12 ounces top round sirloin steak
- 1 Tbsp low-sodium soy sauce
- 2 ounces freshly squeezed lime juice
- 2 Tbsp grapeseed oil
- 2 medium red bell peppers
- 2 medium yellow bell peppers
- 1 medium orange bell pepper
- 1 large white onion
- 1/2 cup of Picante sauce
- 3 ounces white cheddar cheese shredded
- 1/4 cup of fresh cilantro finely chopped
- Sour cream

INSTRUCTIONS

1. In a shallow container, mix soy sauce and lime juice. Place steak in the container and allow to marinate for about 1 hour in the refrigerator.
2. Meanwhile, wash and cut bell peppers half vertically (top to bottom). Take seeds and diaphragms. Slice the peppers in thin strips into one red bell; repeat with yellow pepper.

Slice each half of the remaining yellow, red, and orange peppers and leave four bits of each coloured pepper.

3. Peel and slice in half the onion, then cut into thin strips per half.
4. Place the peppers on a sheet cut side up. Place a tea cubicle of Picante sauce in each pepper and reserve it.
5. Heat oil over medium heat in a cast-iron pot. Add steak to the pan and cook on each side for 2 minutes to hit medium-rare. (If you like more cooked steaks, add one. Remove the steak and place it on a cutting board extra minute to each side's cooking time.). Enable to rest at least 10 minutes before thinly cutting against the grain.
6. Heat the oven to 375 degrees F.
7. Return skillet to medium heat as steak rests. Add additional oil if needed. When the oil is heated, add sliced onions and sliced peppers, and saute for 5-6 minutes until the pepper is soft and onion is translucent.
8. On top of a Picante sauce, add some pepper/onion mixture and top with a few slices of steak and some shredded cheese.
9. Bake, 8-10 minutes or until cheese is bubbly and melted at 375.
10. Remove from oven and serve with cilantro and sour cream.

NUTRITION INFO

Cholesterol: 1mg, Calories: 3kcal

12. CAULIFLOWER PIZZA CRUST

PREP TIME:0 HOURS 15 MINS

TOTAL TIME:0 HOURS 45 MINS

INGREDIENTS

- 1 large roughly chopped head cauliflower
- 1 large egg
- shredded divided mozzarella
- 1/2 cup of freshly grated Parmesan, divided
- kosher salt
- 1/4 cup of marinara
- 2 cloves minced garlic
- 1 cup of halved cherry tomatoes
- Torn fresh basil
- Balsamic glaze

DIRECTIONS

1. Heat the oven to 425 degrees F. Add the cauliflower to one layer and cook to crisp, 3-4 minutes, transfer to clean dish towel (or towels of paper) and squeeze into the bath. In a large pot, bring approximately 1/4" of water to a boil. Add salt.
2. Through the food processor, add drained cauliflower and pulse to grate. Drain excess water in towels.
3. Transfer drained cauliflower to a big bowl, add 1 cup of mozzarella and 1/4 cup of Parmesan, and add salt.
4. Transfer to a bakery plate with cooking spray and pull it into a crust. Bake until golden and dry for 20 minutes.

5. Cover the crust with marinara, remaining mozzarella and Parm, garlic, tomatoes, and bake for 10 minutes more until cheese is melted and crusty.
6. Garnish with basil and balsamic glaze drizzle.

13. SUGAR-FREE PUMPKIN CHEESECAKE MOUSSE

prep time: 10 MINUTES

total time: 10 MINUTES

INGREDIENTS

- 8 ounces softened cream cheese
- 1 cup of canned pumpkin puree
- 1/2 cup of Swerve confectioners sweetener
- 1 tsp pumpkin pie spice
- 1 tsp vanilla extract
- 3/4 cup of heavy whipping cream

DIRECTIONS

1. Beat cream cheese and pumpkin puree together in a mixing bowl with a hand mixer.
2. Add the remaining ingredients and whip for several minutes until smooth, fluffy, and slightly rigid. Don't beat over.
3. Pip into tiny cups and serve.

NUTRITIONAL INFO

Amount Per Serving:

Calories: 255, Protein: 3g Total Carbohydrates: 18g, Sugar Alcohols: 12g, Fiber: 2g, Net Carbohydrates: 4g, Total Fat: 18g

14. SIMPLE TACO SOUP

Prep/Total Time: 25 min.

Ingredients

- 2 pounds ground beef
- 1 envelope taco seasoning
- 1-1/2 cups of water
- 16 ounces undrained mild chilli beans
- 15-1/4 ounces drained whole kernel corn
- 15 ounces pinto beans, rinsed and drained
- 14-1/2 ounces stewed tomatoes
- 10 ounces diced tomato with green chiles
- 4 ounces chopped green chiles
- 1 envelope ranch salad dressing mix

Directions

1. Cook beef in a Dutch oven over medium heat until no pink; drain. Add the taco and blend well. Stir the other ingredients. Bring a boil. Bring a boil. Reduce heat; occasionally stir, uncovered, for 15 minutes or until heated.

Test Kitchen Tips

• If you want, you can make your own taco seasoning for this recipe. Try this combination. Try this blend out.
• The same goes for the blend of the ranch! This is our go-to.

Nutrition Info

370 calories, 7g fibre, 14g fat, 70mg cholesterol, 7g sugars, 1369mg sodium, 35g carbohydrate, 27g protein.

15. MINI HOISIN TURKEY & ZUCCHINI MEATLOAF MUFFINS

Prep Time: 10 minutes

Cook Time: 25 minutes

Total Time: 35 minutes

Ingredients

- 1 1/2 pounds ground turkey
- 1 1/2 cups of grated zucchini liquid squeezed out
- 1/3 cup + 3 tbsp hoisin sauce divided
- 3/4 cup of old-fashioned oats
- 1/4 cup of minced flat-leaf parsley
- 3/4 tsp Chinese 5-spice powder
- 1/2 tsp salt
- 1/2 tsp ground pepper
- 1 egg

Instructions

1. Heat the oven to 350 degrees F. Coat a muffin tin loosely with a cooking spray.
2. Mix turkey, zucchini, 1/3 cup hoisin sauce, oats, parsley, 5-spice powder, salt, pepper, and egg in a big bowl.
3. Use a little less than 1/2 cup of the meatloaf mixture and place each portion in a muffin tin slot.
4. Brush the meatloaves with the 3 tbsp of sauce leftover.
5. On a baking sheet, place the muffin tin. (to catch any drips). Bake for 25 to 30 minutes until the meatloaves are ready. Remove with a small metal spatula, then leave for 10 minutes to rest.

Nutrition Info

Serving: 1Mini Meatloaf | Calories: 118kcal, Carbohydrates: 9g, Calcium: 16mg, Protein: 15g, Fat: 2g, Saturated Fat: 1g, Cholesterol: 45mg, Sodium: 326mg, Vitamin C: 4.5mg, Potassium: 256mg, Fiber: 1g, Sugar: 4g, Vitamin A: 170IU, Iron: 1.1mg

16. SINGLE SERVE BAKED RICOTTA

Prep Time: 5 mins

Cook Time: 20 mins

Total Time: 25 mins

Ingredients

- Olive Oil Spray
- 15- ounce Part-skim ricotta
- ⅓ cup of parmesan cheese
- Basil (⅛ tsp)
- Garlic powder (⅛ tsp)
- • Salt and pepper pinch
- Optional top with marinara sauce smooth

Instructions

1. Heat the oven to 350 degrees F.
2. Spray 5 olive oil ramekins and place on a baking sheet.
3. Combine ricotta, parmesan cheese, basil, garlic powder, salt, and pepper in a medium bowl.
4. Stir the ricotta mixture to combine completely.
5. Place the ricotta mixture into the prepared ramekins in 1/4-1/2 cup.
6. Top with one smooth marinara sauce tbsp.
7. Twenty minutes bake.
8. Serve hot.

Nutrition Info

Serving: 0.33cup,   Calories: 144kcal, Iron: 1mg Carbohydrates: 5g, Protein: 12g, Fat: 8g, Saturated Fat: 5g, Cholesterol: 31mg,

Sugar: 1g, Sodium: 213mg, Potassium: 106mg, Vitamin A: 379IU, Calcium: 310mg

17. BARIATRIC FRIENDLY - CHICKEN CRUST PIZZA

Prep Time: 20m

Cook Time: 20m

Ready In: 40m

Ingredients

- 1 pound ground chicken breast
- 1/2 cup of grated Parmesan cheese
- 1 cup of shredded part-skim mozzarella cheese
- 1/2 tsp garlic powder
- Sea salt and freshly ground black pepper
- Dried oregano
- 1/2 cup of pasta sauce
- Crushed red pepper flakes
- 4 to 5 basil leaves

Instructions

1. Heat the oven to 450 degrees F.
2. Line a baking or pizza pan with parchment paper or foil, sprayed with a spray.
3. The ground chicken with 1/4 cup Parmesan, 1/2 tsp salt, 1/4 tsp powder, 1/2 tsp salt, and 1/2 tsp oregano is mixed in a medium bowl.

4. Transfer the chicken mixture onto the parchment and pat it in a flat rectangle or disc.
5. Cover with a plastic wrap and uniformly press or roll the chicken into or around a 7x10-inch rectangle.
6. Remove the plastic wrap and roast until golden, for 12-15 minutes, draining any liquid that can remain in the pan at 12 minutes.
7. Smear with sauce, scatter with 1/4 cup Parmesan, 3/4 cup Mozzarella, a top layer and sprinkle with crushed red pepper and 1/4 of tsp oregano.
8. Pop back in a hot oven and cook for 10 minutes until melted and bubbly.
9. Sprinkle with chopped basil and remove it from the oven.

Nutrition

Calories 241g, Total Fat - 10.5 g, Saturated Fat - 5.5 g, Protein - 32.6 g Cholesterol - 296.2 mg, Sodium - 455.8 mg, Total Carbohydrate - 3 g, Dietary Fiber - 0.7 g, Calcium - 443.2 mg, Iron - 3.8 mg, Vitamin C - 8.9 mg, Sugars - 1.2 g, Thiamin - 0.1 mg

18. HEALTHY TURKEY LETTUCE WRAPS

Prep Time: 10 mins

Cook Time: 10 mins

Total Time: 20 mins

Ingredients

- 1 pound lean ground turkey
- 1 Tbsp vegetable oil
- 1 small diced onion
- 2 cloves minced garlic
- 1 tsp freshly grated ginger
- 1 bell diced pepper
- 1 Tbsp soy sauce
- 2 Tbsp Oyster Sauce
- 1 tsp sesame oil
- 2 tsp rice vinegar or distilled white vinegar
- 2 green minced onions
- salt, as need
- ground black pepper, as need
- fresh lettuce leaves

Instructions

1. Add oil in a large heated pan. Add onion, garlic, and ginger and cook for translucent cooking.
2. Add turkey to the ground and cook until slightly browned, around 3 minutes. Add soy, hoisin, or oyster, sesame oil, rice vinegar, and add turkey meat.

3. Add bell peppers and green onions and cook around 5 minutes or until all is well combined with turkey. Add salt and pepper as need.
4. You can either serve the filling warmly or let it cool. Serve with salad leaves.

Nutrition Info

Calories: 206kcal, Carbohydrates: 7g, Protein: 28g, Fat: 7g, Saturated Fat: 3g, Cholesterol: 62mg, Sodium: 441mg, Potassium: 458mg, Fiber: 1g, Sugar: 4g, Vitamin A: 1020IU, Vitamin C: 40.4mg, Calcium: 14mg

19. HERBED PEA PUREE AND RICOTTA SALAD WITH BLACK GARLIC AND LEMON CONFITURE

Active: 1 hr 30 mins

Total: 2 hrs 30 mins

Ingredient
Lemon Confiture

- ¾ cup of water
- ¾ cup of sugar
- ½ tsp kosher salt
- 2 firm lemons
- Pea Puree
- ¼ cup of extra-virgin olive oil
- ½ onion

- Kosher salt
- 1 cup of peas
- 2 tbsp mint
- 2 tbsp parsley
- ½ cup of fresh ricotta
- 2 tbsp freshly grated Parmigiano-Reggiano cheese

Salad

- 1 ½ tbsp extra-virgin olive oil
- 12 cloves black garlic
- 1 cup of English peas
- ¼ pound sugar snap peas
- ¼ pound snow peas
- Kosher salt

• Shootings of a pea, radishes, small mint leaves, finely chopped chives, sliced Marcona, and edible flowers.

Directions

Make the Lemon Confiture

1. Heat the oven to 350 degrees F. In a small casserole, mix water, sugar, and salt and bring to boil, stirring to dissolve the sugar. Transfer to small baking and add the lemon slices uniformly. Bake until rinds are translucent and the lemons tender for 20 to 25 minutes. Let cool totally.

Meanwhile, Make the Puree

2. Heat the olive oil in a medium skillet. Add onions, season with salt, and cook over moderate heat, and often stir until brown begins, around 7 minutes. Stir in the peas and cook until heated, around 3 minutes. Stir in the mint and

the parsley for 1 minute until wilted. Shift the mix into a mini food processor and cool fully, then smoothly purée. In a medium bowl, scrape the pea puree and fold into ricotta and Parmigiano-Reggiano. Season to salt.

Prepare the Salad

3. Brush with olive oil a large square of wax paper lightly. Arrange 3 inches away from the black garlic cloves and put another piece of waxed paper on top. Using a rolling pin, roll the cloves gently until they are very flat. Glide the paper onto a plate and freeze about 15 minutes until slightly firm.
4. Meanwhile, blanch English peas, snaps, and snow peas in a large saucepan of salted boiling water for about 3 minutes. Drain, transfer to a bowl, and blend with 1 1/2 olive oil tbsp. Coarsely chop 8 slices of lemon and fold into them—salt season.
5. Scoop on the plates 1/3-cup mounds of the pea puree and spoon warm peas. Peel out the top sheet of wax paper and lay 2 garlic cloves on each mound of pea puree with a small offset spatula. Arrange 1 slice of garlic lemon jam and garnish the salads with pea shoots, radishes, little mint leaves, chives, almonds, and edible flowers. Serve immediately.

Notes

- Black garlic, with a sweet, molasses-like taste, is fermented. It is available in food shops and on blackgarlic.com.

20. HEALTHY CHICKEN BURGERS (LOW-CARB & PALEO)

PREP TIME: 10 minutes

COOK TIME: 10 minutes

TOTAL TIME: 20 minutes

INGREDIENTS

- 1 pound ground chicken
- 1/2 cup of finely diced onion
- 2 cloves minced garlic
- 3/4 tsp fine sea salt
- 1/4 tsp smoked paprika
- freshly ground black pepper

INSTRUCTIONS

1. Mix the chicken, onion, garlic, salt, paprika, and many black pepper grinds into a large bowl. Divide the mixture into 4 even sections so you can shape patties using a spoon.
2. Wet your hands to make dealing with the mixture simpler (it doesn't stick to wet hands and make a burger patty by rubbing it between your hands. Repeat the remaining mixture until 4 evenly-sized patties are approximately 1 inch thick.
3. Grate the olive oil in a 12-inch skillet and place it on the stove over medium-high heat. k Arrange all four chicken burgers on the skillet and allow 5 minutes to cook them. Turn burgers over and cook for 4 to 5 minutes on the other hand, or when tested with a thermometer, until the

burgers reach an internal temperature of 165 degrees F. (You should cut only one in half to make sure that the middle isn't pink too.)

4. Serve your favourite toppings warmly in the grilled burgers. A bun or lettuce wrap can be used! Cooked burgers are maintained in an airtight container to the fridge for up to 3 days or can be frozen for up to 3 months.

NUTRITION INFORMATION

Calories: 173kcal, Carbohydrates: 2g, Protein: 20g, Fat: 9g, Saturated Fat: 3g, Cholesterol: 98mg, Sodium: 505mg, Potassium: 621mg, Fiber: 1g, Sugar: 1g, Vitamin A: 60IU, Vitamin C: 2mg, Calcium: 14mg, Iron: 0.9mg

Recipe Notes:

- You can use turkey rather than chicken if you can find it easier.
- If you follow the rules of the food mix, this recipe is listed as animal protein and can be eaten on a salad or as a salad bowl. (It also makes it low-carbon and nice to keto!)
- Please leave a comment below to let me know how you find this recipe if you try. And if you make any substitutes, please let me know how this works for you too! We will all benefit from your experience.

21. CHEESY CHICKEN BROCCOLI BAKE

PREP TIME: 5 MINS

COOK TIME: 30 MINS

TOTAL TIME: 35 MINS

INGREDIENTS

- 1 tbsp. extra-virgin olive oil
- 1 cup of chopped small yellow onion
- 2 cloves minced garlic
- 1 pound boneless, skinless chicken breasts, cut into 1-inch pieces
- Kosher salt
- Freshly ground black pepper
- 1 cup of white rice
- 2 1/2 cup of divided low-sodium chicken broth
- 1 cup of heavy cream
- 2 cup of broccoli florets
- 1 cup of shredded cheddar
- 1/4 cup of panko bread crumbs

DIRECTIONS

1. 1. Heat oil over medium-high heat in a large oven-safe pot. Add onion and cook, stirring, 5 minutes until soft. Add garlic and cook until fragrant for 1 minute longer. Add chicken and salt and pepper to season. Cook, occasionally stirring, about 6 minutes more until golden.
2. Incorporate rice, heavy cream, and 1 cup of broth. Cook until the rice is soft, about 15 minutes. Include remaining 1/2 cups of broth, broccoli, cheddar cheese, and cook until smooth and melty broccoli, around 10 minutes.

3. Hot broiler. Heat broiler. Sprinkle with bread crumbs and season with salt and pepper in a chicken mixture. Broil for about 2 minutes until golden and crisps.

22. CHICKEN WITH CREAMY MUSHROOM SAUCE

prep time: 10 MINUTES

cook time: 40 MINUTES

total time: 50 MINUTES

INGREDIENTS:

- 8 bone-in, skin-on chicken thighs
- Kosher salt and freshly ground black pepper, as need
- 2 tbsp unsalted butter
- 2 tbsp chopped fresh parsley leaves

FOR THE MUSHROOM SAUCE

- 1 tbsp unsalted butter
- 2 cloves minced garlic
- 8 ounces cremini thinly sliced mushrooms
- 2 tbsp all-purpose flour
- 1 1/2 cups of half and half*
- 1/2 tsp dried thyme
- 1/2 tsp dried basil
- Pinch of crushed red pepper flakes
- Kosher salt and freshly ground black pepper, as need

DIRECTIONS:

1. Heat the oven to 400 degrees F. Cover the 9 to 13 baking platter with nonstick spray lightly.
2. Season salt and pepper chicken thighs to taste.
3. Melt 2 tbsp of butter on medium heat in a large skillet. Add the chicken, skin-side down, sear both sides, about 2-3 minutes per side until golden brown.
4. Place the chicken on the skin in one layer in the prepared baking. Set in oven and roast for about 25-30 minutes, until fully cooked, to an inner temperature of 175 degrees F. Excess drain fat.
5. Melt the remaining tbsp butter in the pot to make the mushroom sauce. Add garlic and champagne and cook, occasionally stirring, about 5-6 minutes until browned and tender.
6. Whisk in flour, around 1 minute, until lightly browned. Gradually whisk halfway through thyme, basil, and crushed flakes of red pepper; Salt and pepper season as need. Cook, whisking continuously, about 3-4 minutes until slightly thickened.
7. Serve chicken with mushroom sauce immediately, garnished with parsley if necessary.

NOTES:

- Half and half of both milk and cream are equal parts. You can replace 3/4 cup of whole milk + 1/4 cup of heavy cream, or 2/3 cup skims of low-fat milk + 1/3 cup of heavy cream for 1 and a half cup.

Nutrition Facts

- Amount Per Serving
- Calories 270.7Calories from Fat 189
- Total Fat 21.0g
- Saturated Fat 8.9g
- Trans Fat 0.2g
- Cholesterol 87.0mg
- Sodium 76.8mg
- Total Carbohydrate 4.6g
- Dietary Fiber 0.4g
- Sugars 0.7g
- Protein 15.9g

23. BANANERBERRY SMOOTHIE

Prep: 10 mins

Total: 10 mins

Ingredients

- 1 cup of fresh strawberries
- 1 banana sliced
- 1 cup of fresh peaches
- 1 cup of apples
- 1 ½ cups of vanilla ice cream
- 1 ½ cups of ice cubes
- ½ cup of milk

Directions

1. Mix strawberries, bananas, peaches, apples, and ice cream in a blender. Mix until it's smooth. Add ice, pour in the milk, and smoothly blend again. Serve instantly.

Nutrition Info

Per Serving:

cholesterol 48.4mg, 354 calories, fat 12.6g, Protein 6.8g, carbohydrates 57.8g, sodium 108.7mg.

24. BACON CHEESEBURGER MEATBALLS

PREP TIME: 5 minutes

COOK TIME: 25 minutes

TOTAL TIME: 30 minutes

INGREDIENTS

- Farm Rich Original Meatballs
- American Cheese, cut into small pieces
- Pre-Cooked Bacon slices, cut into small pieces.
- Ice Berg Lettuce, cut into small pieces.
- Grape Tomatoes, cut in half
-

INSTRUCTIONS

2. Bake as many original Farm Rich meatballs as you like and follow the instructions in the box.
3. Break small pieces of American cheese into Meanwhile
4. Melton top when baked meatballs.

5. 5. Stack your favourite toppings for toothpicks. I've been wearing bacon, some iceberg lettuce, and a half grape tomato.
6. When the baking time is finished, top and meatball with a small slice of cheese, bring it back into the oven, and let it melt for a few minutes.
7. Poke the stacked skewer into the meatball, plate, and serve.
8. Serve "sauce" with ketchup, mayo, and mustard if desired.

NUTRITION INFO:

Amount Per Serving: CALORIES: 38TOTAL FAT: 3g; SATURATED FAT: 1g; TRANS FAT: 0g; UNSATURATED FAT: 2g; CHOLESTEROL: 9mg; SODIUM: 103mg; CARBOHYDRATES: 1g; FIBER: 0g; SUGAR: 1g; PROTEIN: 2g

25. SPAGHETTI SQUASH BOATS

Total Time

Prep: 1 hour

Bake: 20 min.

Ingredients

- 1 medium spaghetti squash
- 1/4 pound ground beef
- 1/2 cup of chopped onion
- 1/2 cup of chopped green pepper
- 1/2 cup of sliced fresh mushrooms
- 1 garlic minced clove
- 1/2 tsp dried basil
- 1/2 tsp dried oregano
- 1/4 tsp salt
- 1/8 tsp pepper
- 14-1/2 ounces drained diced tomatoes
- 1/3 cup of shredded part-skim mozzarella cheese

Directions

1. Half the squash, scoop out seeds. Place squash in baking cut down the side. Fill with hot water at 1/2 in depth. Bake, uncovered, 30-40 minutes or tenderly at 375 degrees F.
2. If you're cool enough to handle, scoop squash and separate strands with a bucket; set shells and squash aside.
3. Cook beef, onion, and green pepper on medium heat in a skillet until the meat are not rose any more; rinse. Add

champagne, garlic, basil, oregano, salt, and pepper; mix and cook for two minutes. Cook and stir for 2 minutes. Add tomatoes. Delete in squad "Stack" your preferred toppings on toothpicks.

4. Cook, uncovered, about ten minutes before liquid evaporates. Fill shells; put in the flake bakery tray.
5. 5. Bake, uncovered, at 350 degrees for 15 minutes. Bake for 5 minutes or until the cheese is melted. Cheese.

26. EASY BAKED FALAFEL

Prep Time: 10 minutes

Cook Time: 24 minutes

Total Time: 34 minutes

INGREDIENTS

- 1 15 ounces can chickpeas, drained and rinsed
- 1/4 cup of chopped onion
- 3 cloves fresh garlic
- 1/2 cup of fresh parsley
- 1 Tbsp avocado oil
- 2 tsp lemon juice
- 1 tsp ground cumin
- 1 tsp ground coriander
- Sea salt (3/4 tsp)
- Cayenne pinch
- Baking soda (1/2 tsp)
- 3 Tbsp oat flour
- avocado oil cooking spray

INSTRUCTIONS

1. Heat the oven to 375 degrees F. Spray a baking sheet with oil.
2. In a food processor, add the pulse, chickpeas, onion, garlic, oil, parsley, lemon juice, cumin, coriander, cayenne, and salt until mixed. Or you could end up with hummus. You don't want to overprocess the mixture. Moreover, with a few chickpeas, the falafel gives a good texture. Mix the baking soda and the oatmeal. Your mixture should hold very well at this stage.
3. Scoop spoonfuls into tiny pieces of mixture; you should get 15. Place on the baker's prepared pan.
4. Bake for 10 to 12 minutes or until falafel is golden and cooked through for another 10 to 12 minutes.

NUTRITION

Serving Size: Protein: 6g, 3 falafel, Calories: 143, Carbohydrates: 24g, Sugar: 1g, Sodium: 648mg, Fiber: 6g Fat: 5g.

27. HEALTHY MEXICAN PIZZA

READY IN: 14mins

INGREDIENTS

- 2whole wheat tortillas
- 1/4cup of pureed black beans
- 1/4cup of Sliced tomatoes
- 1/4cup of Sliced bell pepper
- 1/4cup of canned corn
- 1/4cup of spinach leaves
- 1tsp oregano
- 1/4cup of Sliced mango
- 1/2cup of salsa
- 1/4cup of Mexican shredded blend cheese
- 1/4cup of cottage cheese

DIRECTIONS

1. Heat the oven to 350 degrees F.
2. Tomatoes slice, bell peppers, and mangoes.
3. Stack tortillas and bake them for a few minutes or up to crispy for 350 minutes.
4. Add spinach leaves on top of the beans with a food processor with pure black beans on the tortilla, and add pineapple/mango, sliced vegetables, corn, and salsa.
5. Sprinkle all the cheese and oregano, put it back and bake for 10-12 minutes or until the cheese is melted and the pizza is heated. Cool salsa and cottage cheese are available.

28. THE BEST TOFU SCRAMBLE

cook time: 10 MINUTES

total time: 10 MINUTES

Ingredients

- 1 tbsp olive oil
- 16-ounce block firm tofu
- 2 tbsp nutritional yeast
- 1/2 tsp salt, or more as need
- 1/4 tsp turmeric
- 1/4 tsp garlic powder
- 2 tbsp non-dairy milk, unsweetened and unflavored

Instructions

1. Heat olive oil in a saucepan over medium heat. Mash the tofu block with a pan or a fork right in the pan. You can also crumble it with your hands into the pan. Cook, frequently stirring, 3-4 minutes until most of the tofu water is gone.
2. Add the powder of nutrient yeast, salt, turmeric, and garlic. Cook and stir for about 5 minutes constantly.
3. Into the pan, pour non-dairy milk and stir to blend. Serve with sliced avocado, sauce, parsley, steam, toast, or any other breakfast item immediately. Serve immediately.

Notes

- Tofu Scramble is also good with all kinds of mixed-in vegetables. Plants for adding before tofu: 1/4 cup diced onion or a few cloves of minced garlic. Sprinkle 2-3 minutes in oil before adding and pulling the tofu. Fresh spinach, kale, thin sliced red peppers, tiny broccoli, or fresh spliced and spicy tomatoes. Add these to the tofu after adding the milk and cook for a few minutes.

- Omit the oil if the tofu scramble oil is desired.
- You can use every kind of milk you like, such as soy, almond, cashew, oat, or coconut milk. Make sure it is unflavored and non-sweetened.

Nutrition

serving: 1serving, calories: 288kcal, carbohydrates: 9g, protein: 24g, fat: 18g, saturated fat: 2g, sodium: 600mg, potassium: 168mg, fiber: 4g, sugar: 1g, vitamin a: 31iu, calcium: 302mg, iron: 3mg

29. VEGAN CAESAR SALAD WITH CRISPY TOFU CROUTONS

Prep Time: 10 mins

Cook Time: 20 mins

Total Time: 30 minutes

Ingredients

- 8 cups of chopped romaine

Dressing

- ½ cup of soaked raw cashews
- ¼ cup of coconut milk, canned + whole
- 2 Tbsp water
- 1 Tbsp white wine vinegar
- 1 Tbsp lemon juice
- 1 Tbsp tamari
- 1 Tbsp nutritional yeast
- 1 tsp sea salt
- 1 tsp black pepper
- Dash of cayenne

Tofu

- 2 Tbsp olive oil
- 1 block extra firm tofu
- 1 Tbsp Italian seasoning blend
- ½ tsp sea salt
- ½ tsp black pepper

Instructions

1. Wash and dry Romaine, then chop in a big bowl. One with a lid, preferably! Nice until later. Cool.
2. Combine all ingredients for Caesar dressing in a food processor or blender. Pulse until creamy and smooth. If it's too thick, add a little more water to thin your liking. I love the thick cohesiveness! Set aside at a later date.
3. Drain tofu and press to remove the excess water as much as possible. Cut the tofu into cubes around 1" square – or any size that you want to have croutons! Add 1 table sponge of olive oil, Italian seasoning, sea salt, and pepper to the chopped tofu into a ziplock bag (or large bowel). Toss to combine. Toss to combine.
4. Heat 1 tbsp of olive oil to medium in a large nonstick or cast-iron skillet. Fill in tofu and let the cubes get a good sear. Cook for a total of 15-20 minutes, and sometimes brown the tofu. Enter the pot and allow it to cool.
5. When tofu is cool, add tofu to the roman bowl and pour over the dressing. Mix thoroughly until it is well hidden. Serve and have fun!

30. VEGETARIAN CHILI

prep time: 20 minutes

cook time: 30 minutes

total time: 50 minutes

INGREDIENTS

- 2 tbsp olive oil
- 1 small diced yellow onion

- 1 tbsp minced garlic
- 1 red diced bell pepper
- 2 tbsp ground chilli powder
- 1/2 tbsp dried oregano
- 1 tsp ground cumin
- 1/2 tsp EACH: dried basil, seasoned salt, cayenne pepper, paprika
- 1/4 tsp cracked pepper
- 1/2 tbsp white sugar
- 14.5 ounces EACH fire-roasted diced tomatoes
- 14.5 ounces EACH black beans, drained and rinsed
- 14.5 ounces pinto beans, drained and rinsed
- 4 ounces fire-roasted diced green chiles
- 1 cup of frozen corn
- 1 cup of vegetable stock
- 1 bay leaf
- 2 tbsp fresh lime juice
- Toppings: cheddar cheese, fat-free sour cream, avocado, cilantro, chives, tortilla strips, etc.

INSTRUCTIONS

1. Place on medium heat a big heavy-bottomed pot (or dutch oven). Pour in the olive oil and wait about 20 seconds to shimmer. Add onion diced and stir for 3-4 minutes. Add the dizzy pepper and cook these vegetables until they are all very soft, stirring periodically for 6-9 minutes.

2. Thin all your spices and blend them into a small bowl: chilli powder, oregano, cumin, dried basil, salt, cayenne pepper, paprika, pepper, and sucre while the vegetables become soft. Stir and reserve until the onion/pepper is soft.

3. Add the garlic and all the seasonings that you measured already and reserve. Stir constantly, cook until seasonings and garlic are odorous, about 45 seconds - 1 minute.
4. Carefully add tomatoes into the UNDRAINED (they can sizzle a bit) and stir. Add the drained and rinsed black beans, pinto beans, chillies (if required), frozen maize, and vegetable stocks. Drained and rinsed. Add the leaf to the harbour.
5. Stir to merge it all. Reduce heat as necessary to hold a gentle stirring for 25-30 minutes, and stir occasionally.
6. Remove 1 and 1/2 chilli cups and turn to the mixer. To prevent a mess, insert the centre of your blender lid and keep your kitchen towel tightly over the top. Sure that the lid is tightly modelled and combined with the towel. Pour this mixture back into your chilli until smooth. Remove to merge.
7. Add fresh lime and cilantro as you like—taste season (I always add in a little bit more salt & pepper). Garnish with everybody's favourite toppings individual bowls. Acid cream and cheddar cheese are a must for us!

RECIPE NOTES

- Spiciness: depending on the actual spices that you use (some brands are hotter/milder than others you would want spices in this chilli to scale up or down.

NUTRITION INFO

Calories: 264kcal

31. VEGGIE-TURKEY BURGERS

Total: 35 min

Ingredients

- ½ cup of finely shredded carrot
- ¼ cup of soft whole wheat bread crumbs
- ¼ cup of thinly sliced green onions
- 2 tbsp milk
- ¼ tsp dried Italian seasoning, crushed
- ¼ tsp garlic salt
- Dash cayenne pepper
- 12 ounces lean ground turkey or chicken
- Nonstick cooking spray
- ¼ cup of Dijon-style mustard
- ½ tsp curry powder
- 4 whole wheat or white hamburger buns, split and toasted
- Lettuce leaves
- Shredded or thinly sliced zucchini
- Sliced tomato

Directions

1. Combine the first seven ingredients in a medium bowl (through cayenne pepper). Add turkey ground; blend well. Mix in four 1/2-inch-thick patties. Shape.
2. Coat the cooking spray in the grill pan; heat over medium heat. Add patties, cook for 10-13 minutes or until pink (165°F) is no more, and turn once.
3. In the meantime, mix the mustard with the curry powder.

4. Fill buns of burger and lettuce, zucchini, tomato, and mustard mixture if needed.

Nutrition Info

Per Serving:

260 calories, calcium 143mg, total fat 9g, saturated fat 2g, vitamin b12 1mcg, polyunsaturated fat 2g, thiamin 0mg, monounsaturated fat 3g, cholesterol 64mg, sodium 703mg, potassium 269mg, carbohydrates 25g, fibre 3g, sugar 5g, vitamin b6 0mg, riboflavin 0mg, protein 21g, trans fatty acid 0g, vitamin a 2687IU, vitamin c 2mg, thiamin 0mg, niacin equivalents 7mg, folate 15mcg, iron 2mg.

32. HONEY GINGER CHICKEN STIR FRY

Prep: 10 minutes

Cook: 15 minutes

Total: 25 minutes

INGREDIENTS
Chicken Stir Fry

- 16 ounces boneless, skinless chicken breasts, cut into chunks
- 1.5 tbsp avocado oil
- 1 tbsp minced garlic
- 8 cups of broccoli florets
- 1/2 cup of shredded carrots

Sauce

- 1/4 cup of honey
- 1/4 cup of low-sodium soy sauce

- 1 tbsp grated fresh ginger
- 1 tsp sriracha
- 1 tbsp hoisin sauce
- 2 tbsp water
- 2 tsp cornstarch

INSTRUCTIONS

1. 1. Heat avocado oil in a wide pan over medium/high heat. Add chicken breast to the pan and cook for 2-3 minutes when oil is fragrant.
2. Prepare the sauce by whisking all the ingredients together until most cornstarch is dissolved. Set aside. Set aside.
3. Then add remaining stir fry (except carrots) ingredients and sprinkle for a couple of minutes before adding the sauce. Bring to a boil the sauce and reduce to low, add carrots, and let it cool six to eight minutes.
4. Take the heat and serve with white rice, brown rice, or quinoa!

TIPS & NOTES

- In nutrition information, rice is no Place the zucchini in a large pott included.

NUTRITION INFORMATION

Serving:

Size: 1/4 Calories: 305, Cholesterol: 34 Sugar: 20 Fat: 9 Fiber: 5 Protein: 28 Carbohydrates: 34

33. MEATLESS ZUCCHINI LASAGNA

Total Time

Prep: 45 min.

Bake: 30 min. + standing

Ingredients

- 6 lasagna noodles
- 1 medium chopped onion
- 2 tsp olive oil
- 2 garlic minced cloves
- 2 cups of water
- 6 ounces each tomato paste
- 2-1/2 tsp each dried thyme, basil, and oregano
- 3/4 tsp salt
- 3 medium thinly sliced zucchini
- 1 large lightly beaten egg
- 15 ounces part-skim ricotta cheese
- 2 cups of shredded part-skim mozzarella cheese
- 1/4 cup of grated Parmesan cheese

Directions

1. Cook noodles according to the instructions of the box. Meanwhile, saute onion in oil softly in a large nonstick skillet. Cook the garlic 1 minute longer. Add garlic. Stir in sugar, paste with tomato and seasonings. Bring to boil. Bring to boil. Reduce heat; cover and cook for 10 minutes.
2. 2. Place the zucchini in a big pot; add 1/2 in. Water. Water. Bring to boil. Bring to boil. Reduce heat; cook for 5 minutes: drain and reserve. Combine egg and ricotta cheese in a small bowl.

3. Drain noodle. Drain noodles. In a 13x9-in position, 1/2 cup of tomato sauce. Coated bakery with spray cooking; top with three noodles. Layer with half a mixture of ricotta and zucchini. Cover with half of the remainder of the tomato sauce and 1 cup of mozzarella. Over and over again, layers.
4. Cover and bake for 25 minutes at 375 degrees F. Sprinkle with Parmesan cheese. Uncover. Bake for 5-10 minutes, or bubble up. Enable 10 minutes to stand before cutting.

Nutrition Info

1 piece: 272 calories, 28g carbohydrate, 10g fat, 55mg cholesterol, 28g carbohydrate, 454mg sodium, 18g protein.

34. CURRIED BUTTERNUT SQUASH SOUP

PREP TIME: 5 minutes

COOK TIME: 25 minutes

TOTAL TIME: 30 minutes

Ingredients
SOUP

- 1 Tbsp coconut oil
- 2 medium shallots
- 2 cloves minced garlic
- 6 cups of peeled & chopped butternut squash
- 1 pinch each sea salt + black pepper
- 1/4 tsp ground cinnamon
- 1 14-ounce can light coconut milk
- 2 cups of vegetable broth

- 1-3 Tbsp maple syrup
- 1-2 tsp chilli garlic

Optional

- Toasted seeds of pumpkin
- Chilli paste garlic.
- Full fat coconut milk

Instructions

1. Over medium heat, heat a large pot.
2. Add oil, shallots, and garlic once warmed. Saute for 2 minutes, stirring sometimes.
3. Add the butternut squash and season with salt, pepper, cinnamon, and curry powder. Stir to coat—cover and cook, stirring for 4 minutes occasionally.
4. Add coconut milk, vegetable broth, maple syrup or cocoon sugar, and chilli pepper (optional - heat).
5. Bring to a low boil over medium heat and reduce heat to low, cover and cook for 15 minutes or until the squash of butternut is tender.
6. Using an immersion blender or transfer soup to the blender and puree until smooth and creamy. If a blender is used, return the soup to the pot.
7. Change the seasonings and add additional curry powder, salt, or sweetener as required. Continue cooking over medium heat for a few more minutes.
8. Serve as is or with choice garnishes (options above). Mind to store leftovers in a refrigerator for 3-4 days or up to 1 month in a freezer. Best when cool.

Notes

- Inspired by my Quick Soup Pumpkin and Sweet Spicy Curry Soupe Pumpkin.
- Nutrition information is a rough approximation measured using coconut oil with less maple syrup and no toppings.

Nutrition

Serving: 1 servings; Carbohydrates: 48.8 g; Calories: 287; Protein: 5.1 g; Trans Fat: 0 g; Fat: 11 g; Saturated Fat: 8 g; Polyunsaturated Fat: 0.35 g; Monounsaturated Fat: 0.9 g; Cholesterol: 0 mg; Calcium: 180 mg; Sodium: 287 mg; Potassium: 1123 mg; Vitamin C: 72.6 mg; Fiber: 12.4 g; Sugar: 15.1 g; Vitamin A: 35550 IU; Iron: 3.8 mg

35. SHRIMP GAZPACHO

Total Time

Prep: 15 min. + chilling

Ingredients

- 6 cups of spicy hot V8 juice
- 2 cups of cold water
- 1/2 cup of lime juice
- 1/2 cup of minced fresh cilantro
- 1/2 tsp salt
- 1/4 to 1/2 tsp hot pepper sauce
- 1 pound peeled and deveined cooked shrimp tails removed
- 1 medium seeded and diced cucumber
- 2 medium seeded and chopped tomatoes

- 2 medium peeled and chopped ripe avocados

Directions

1. Mix the first 6 ingredients in a large non-reactive bowl. Stir the remaining ingredients carefully. Cool, sealed, 1 hour before serving.

Nutrition Information

1 cup: 10g protein, 112 calories, 57mg cholesterol, 399mg sodium, 4g fat, 9g carbohydrate.

36. EASY ONE-PAN ROASTED SHRIMP AND VEGGIES

Prep Time: 10 minutes

Cook Time: 20 minutes

Total Time: 30 minutes

Ingredients

- 1 lb shrimp raw
- 2 cups of broccoli florets
- 1 zucchini cubed
- 1/2 onion cubed
- 1 bell pepper cubed
- 1 medium carrot thinly sliced
- 2 tbsp olive oil

Seasoning mix

- 1 tsp salt
- 1 tsp Italian seasoning
- 1/4 tsp paprika

- 1/4 tsp black pepper

Instructions

2. Heat the oven to 425 degrees F. for at least 10 minutes, line a large foil sheet, and set aside.
3. Place veggies and sprinkle with half the seasoning mixture and 1 tbsp of oil in a wide bowl. Combine shrimp, the remainder of the savoury mixture (half), and 1 tbsp oil in another bowl; set aside shrimp.
4. In the grill, pour the veggies and cook for 12-15 minutes or until slightly chopped. Add shrimp and cook for 5 minutes or tenderly pink. Take off the oven and enjoy hot rice, pasta, or salads!

37. FALL HARVEST HOMEMADE VEGETABLE SOUP

Prep Time: 30 minutes

Cook Time: 45 minutes

Total Time: 1 hour 15 minutes

Ingredients

- 3 tbsp olive oil
- 4 cloves garlic minced
- 1 yellow onion diced
- 3 celery stalks sliced
- 3 carrots sliced
- 3 parsnips sliced
- 2 sweet potatoes cubed peeled
- 2 cups of sweet peppers chopped sliced

- 28 ounces diced tomatoes undrained
- 15 ounces rinsed garbanzo beans drained
- 1 cup of spinach chopped
- 4 cups of vegetable broth
- 4 - 6 cups of water
- 3 bay leaves
- 1 tsp dried Italian seasoning
- 1 tsp salt
- 1/2 tsp dried thyme
- 1/2 tsp black pepper

Instructions

1. 1. Heat oil with medium-high heat in a large pot. Add garlic, onion, celery, carrots, parsnips, sweet potatoes, and peppers. Cook and stir, constantly stirring for 10 - 15 minutes.
2. Mix the undrained tomatoes. Add the beans of garbanzo.
3. Pour over the vegetables, the vegetable broth, and the water. Mix in the bay leaves, salt, and pepper. Season.
4. Add the spinach chopped, stir and bring to a low boil. Reduce fire, cover, and cover, or until vegetables are tender for 45 minutes.
5. As needed, taste and re-season. Hot Serve.

Nutrition

Serving: 1cup | Calories: 174kcal, Calcium: 78mg, Carbohydrates: 29g, Protein: 5g, Sugar: 9g Fat: 4g, Saturated Fat: 0g, Cholesterol: 0mg, Sodium: 554mg, Vitamin C: 48.3mg, Potassium: 604mg, Fiber: 7g, Vitamin A: 6930IU, Iron: 2.4mg

38. ALMOND CRUSTED CHICKEN TENDERS

PREP TIME: 15 MIN

COOK TIME: 20 MIN

TOTAL TIME: 35 MIN

Ingredients

- 1 lb boneless skinless chicken breast, cut into strips
- 1/2 cup of almond meal
- 1/2 tsp paprika
- 1/2 tsp garlic powder
- 1/2 tsp onion powder
- Salt (1/2 tsp)
- Pepper (1/2 tsp)
- Cumin (1/2 tsp)
- 1 egg
- 1 egg white

Instructions

1. Heat the oven to 375 degrees F. Line an aluminium foil bake and place a wire rack on it.
2. Mix the almond flour, paprika, garlic powder, onion powder, salt, and cumin. Mix. In a shallow dish, whisk the egg and egg white together.
3. Then wash the chicken into the egg and press into the meal of the almond. Place on the rack of wire. Bake for 20 minutes until cooked halfway through.

Nutritional Information

Serving Size: 2 tenders

Amount Per Serving

Calories from Fat 84

Calories 233

Total Fat 10g

Saturated Fat 1g

Monounsaturated Fat 0g

Cholesterol 102mg

Polyunsaturated Fat 0g

Sodium 368mg

Total Carbohydrate 4g

Dietary Fiber 2g

Sugars 1g

Protein 30g

39. CRUSTLESS CHICKEN POT PIE

Prep Time:20 minutes

Cook Time:30 minutes

Total Time:50 minutes

Ingredients

- 2 cups of mashed potatoes boxed
- 1 pound of chicken cooked and diced
- 2 3/4 cups of chicken stock
- 2 cups of frozen mixed vegetables
- 1 cup of shredded sharp cheddar cheese
- 3 tbsp. butter
- 1/3 cup of flour
- salt and pepper as need

Instructions

1. Heat the oven to 400 degrees F.
2. Prepare mashed potatoes or make homemade mashed potatoes.
3. In a wide oven-safe fry pan, melt butter.
4. In flour, whisk into melted butter.
5. In a flour mixture, slowly whisk chicken stock and fry until thickened—season with pepper and salt.
6. Add frozen veggies, shredded cheese, and chicken diced. Bring medium heat to a boil.
7. Dish into eight ramekins
8. Top with potatoes mashed.
9. Thirty minutes Bake.

Nutrition Info

Calories: 350kcal, Calcium: 128mg, Carbohydrates: 25g, Protein: 19g, Sugar: 2g, Fat: 19g, Saturated Fat: 7g, Cholesterol: 60mg, Vitamin A: 2730IU, Sodium: 625mg, Potassium: 474mg, Fiber: 3g, Vitamin C: 18mg, Iron: 2mg

40. ZUCCHINI NOODLES WITH TURKEY MARINARA RECIPE

Total Time: 45 mins

INGREDIENTS
For the Zucchini noodles:

- about 2-3 medium zucchini, cut into noodle strips with a spiralizer
- 1 tbsp olive oil

For the turkey marinara sauce:

- 2 tbsp olive oil
- 1 pound ground turkey
- 1 medium minced onion
- 1 large clove minced garlic
- 14.5 ounces of crushed tomato sauce
- 1/4 tsp dried thyme
- 1/2 tsp paprika
- 1 tsp Worcestershire sauce
- 1/2 tsp ground dry mustard
- 1/2 tsp sugar
- 1/2 tsp kosher, as need

- fresh cracked black pepper, as need
- 1/2 cup of grated parmesan cheese, as need

INSTRUCTIONS

1. Prep the zucchini noodles: Heat a large saucepan over medium to high temperatures. Add 1 tbsp of olive oil and saute the zucchini noodles between 2-3 minutes until tender. Continue to release excess vapour. Do not overcook the zucchini noodles.
2. Make turkey marinara sauce: heat medium to high heat in a medium saucepan. Add olive oil, garlic, and onions. Cook until luscious.
3. Add ground turkey and cook for about 5 minutes, until light brown. If you cook with the remaining cooked turkey, just cook the turkey, about 2-3 minutes, until heated.
4. Add tomato sauce, dried thyme, pepper, Worcestershire sauce, sweet mustard, salt, and pepper.
5. Bring the sauce to medium heat and then cook to low. Cook the sauce for about 20-25 minutes on low heat.
6. Serve the sauce over the noodles of zucchini noodles— Parmesan cheese sprinkle.

41. SPINACH, MUSHROOM & GOAT CHEESE STUFFED PORK LOIN

Prep Time: 15 minutes

Cook Time: 1 hour 15 minutes

Total Time: 1 hour 30 minutes

INGREDIENTS

- 4-5 pounds Boneless Center Cut Pork Loin
- 9 ounces washed Fresh Baby Spinach Leaves
- 1 cup of sliced Mushrooms
- 1 clove chopped Garlic
- 1 cup of Crumbled Goat Cheese
- Kosher Salt as need
- Fresh Ground Black Pepper, to taste
- Garlic Powder, as need
- 1/2 cup of Dry White Wine
- 1/2 cup of Chicken Broth
- Kitchen String

INSTRUCTIONS

1. Into a food processor, add spinach, mushrooms, and garlic and pulse until a paste is made. Take and apply to a bowl, then fold the goat's cheese gently.
2. Trim any extra fat from your roast and "roll cut" your pork off to lie flat. Using a tenderizer, sprinkle the meat gently to ensure even thickness.
3. Layer the mixture uniformly over your meat. Roll the pork away, tie it in the kitchen and place it in the oven in a healthy bakery. Season the salt, pepper, and garlic

powder and add the bottom of the pan of the wine and chicken broth.

4. Bake at 350 degrees F for around 75-90 minutes (subject to total weight) or to the correct internal temperature (I prefer 165 degrees F) every 20 minutes. Remove from the oven and allow 10 minutes to rest. Remove the string and break it into 1" slices.

42. GARLIC GINGER PORK STIR FRY

Prep Time: 10 mins

Cook Time: 10 mins

Total Time: 20 mins

INGREDIENTS
STIR FRY SAUCE

- 1 cup of beef broth
- 2 Tbsp cornstarch
- 3 Tbsp light soy sauce
- 2 tsp dark soy sauce
- 2 Tbsp light brown sugar
- 1/2 - 1 tsp sambal oelek chilli paste
- 1 1/2 tsp fresh ginger - grated
- 1/4 tsp crushed red pepper flakes

STIR FRY

- 1 pound boneless pork chops, sliced into thin strips against the grain
- 2 Tbsp divided vegetable oil
- 4 cloves minced garlic
- 1 1/2 tsp finely minced fresh ginger
- 1 cup of snow peas

- 1/2 cup of shredded carrots
- 1 cup of sliced mushrooms
- a drizzle of toasted sesame oil
- minced fresh cilantro
- green onions, chopped
- peanuts crushed
- 8 - 12 ounces Hokkien stir fry noodles

INSTRUCTIONS:

MAKE THE SAUCE

1. Combine maize starch and broth in a small bowl until smooth. Add soja sauces, brown sugar, sambal oelek, ginger, and red pepper flakes.

MAKE THE STIR FRY

1. In a wok or large skillet, stir-fry pork in 1 tbsp of oil and heat for 2-3 minutes over MED-HIGH until browned. Remove to aboard. Remove.
2. Add 1 tbsp of oil, garlic, and ginger in the same pan. Cook for 30 seconds, then add fried vegetables and cook until crisp.
3. Add the mixture of the broth and the vegetables. Cook and stir until thickened for 1 minute. Add to boil.
4. Add pork and stir fry noodles; heat through. Drizzle with sesame oil, add garnish, and serve.

NOTES

- Pork tenderloin can be replaced if needed for pork chops.
- I want to add a black pepper sprinkle before serving, but that is entirely optional.

43. WILD SALMON COLLARD GREEN WRAPS

PREP TIME: 10mins

COOK TIME: 15mins

INGREDIENTS

- 2 fillets washed and patted dry wild salmon
- Salt
- Black pepper
- 4 large hard stems removed leaves collard greens
- 1/2 cup of hummus
- 1 cup of shredded carrots
- 1 cup of sliced thin cucumber
- 2 halved and sliced avocados
- 1/2 cup of alfalfa sprouts
- 12 spears steamed until tender asparagus

METHOD

1. Heat the oven to 350 degrees F. Season salmon with pepper and salt. Place on a lined baking sheet and bake for 15-18 minutes, until just done. Let it cool and smooth into small bits.
2. Microwave every leaf on a towel of paper one at a time to smooth out. Disseminate hummus in the centre of each leaf. Divide the salmon and disseminate the hummus: spread carrots, cucumbers, avocado, alfalfa sprouts, and asparagus evenly between each leaf.
3. Roll each leaf carefully to create a wrap. Halve to serve.

44. MARYLAND CRAB CAKES RECIPE (LITTLE FILLER)

Prep Time: 40 minutes

Cook Time: 15 minutes

Total Time: 55 minutes

Ingredients

- 1 large egg
- 1/4 cup of mayonnaise
- 1 Tbsp chopped fresh parsley
- 2 tsp dijon mustard
- 2 tsp Worcestershire sauce
- 1 tsp Old Bay seasoning
- 1 tsp fresh lemon juice, add more for serving
- 1/8 tsp salt
- 1 pound fresh lump crab meat
- 2/3 cup of Saltine cracker crumbs
- optional: 2 Tbsp melted salted

Instructions

1. Whisk together in a big bowl the egg, mayonnaise, parsley, dijon mustard, Worcestershire sauce, Old Bay, lemon juice, and salt. Place the crab meat on top, then the cracker crumbs. With a rubber spatula or a large spoon, fold together very gently and carefully. You don't want the crab meat to break up!
2. Cover tightly and cool for at least 30 minutes until 1 day.

3. Heat the oven to 450 degrees F. Grease a rimmed baking sheet generously with butter, spray, or silicone baking mat.
4. Using a 1/2 cup measuring cup, portion the crab cake mixture on the baking sheet to six mounds. Using your hands or your spoon to compact each mound so that no lumps hang or fall apart. (Don't flatten!) Brush each with melted butter for extra flavour.
5. Bake around the edges and on top for 12-14 minutes or until slightly browned. Drizzle with fresh citrus juice and serve wet.
6. Tightly cover the remaining crab cakes and cool for up to 5 days or freeze for up to 3 months.

Notes

- Freezing instructions: Unbaked cakes can be freeze for up to 3 months. Thaw, brush with melted butter and then bake as directed in the refrigerator. Baked and cooled crab cakes can also be freeze for up to 3 months. Thaw, then warm-up for about 10-15 minutes in a 350 degrees F. oven or until all warmed up. Or bake frozen crab cakes for around 25-30 minutes at 350 degrees F.
- What Crab Meat to Use: See Best Crab Meat for Crab Cakes in the blog post above for all questions about which crab to use. I highly recommend lump crab fresh (cooled) seafood.
- Smaller sizes: Split the mixture into 12 1/4 cup pieces for smaller crab cakes. Divide into 24 2 Tbsp size portions for mini crab cakes—Bake at the same temperature of the oven. The baking time for these smaller sizes is shorter. The crab cakes are achieved in mild browning of the tops and edges.

45. BAKED TOMATOES WITH CRAB

READY IN: 30mins

INGREDIENTS

- 1/2cup of finely ground nuts, like pecans
- 2large halved tomatoes
- 1cup of fresh, well-drained lump crabmeat
- 1cup of shredded reduced-fat Monterey jack cheese
- 1/2cup of finely chopped black olives
- 1/2cup of finely chopped mushroom
- 1/2cup of finely chopped parsley
- 1garlic minced clove
- 1/2tsp dried oregano
- 1/2tsp dried basil

DIRECTIONS

1. Heat the oven to 350 degrees F. Coat a spray cooking baking. Place the soil nuts on a plate. Coat with a cooking spray on both sides of the tomato halves. Sprinkle the cut sides into the nuts to cover well. Place the tomatoes on the breadboard.
2. Combine crab meat, cheese, olives, champagne, pillow, garlic, oregano, and basil in a large bowl. Divide the crab mixture between the tomatoes at night. Bake for 15 minutes or bubb4lly until hot.

46. PARMESAN CRUSTED BURGERS WITH GRILLED

Prep Time: 20 minutes

Cook Time: 20 minutes

Total Time: 40 minutes

Ingredients
BURGERS

- 1 pound lean ground beef 500 grams
- 1 egg
- 8 tbsp freshly grated parmesan cheese divided 40 grams
- 3-4 sprigs freshly chopped Italian parsley
- salt and pepper as need

GRILLED VEGGIES

- 1 sliced onion
- 1 big firm sliced ripe tomato
- oregano
- basil
- salt

Instructions
BURGERS

1. Mix ground beef, egg, 3 tbsp of parmesan (15 grams), chopped parsley, salt, and pepper in a medium bowl, and shape into 4 patties.
2. Add 5 tbsp of parmesan cheese (25 grams) and coat with patties one by one in a small dish.
3. Add 1 cubic metal of olive oil to a medium pan, then add patties and cook until no longer pink and browned.

GRILLED VEGGIES

1. Tomato and onion slices on an indoor grill or BBQ grill, drizzle with tomato slices and olive oil, salt, oregano, and basil, and do the same with onions except for basil. Flip over them, repeat them. Grill until cooked. Grill until cooked. There was a mistake (the onion slices will take longer than the tomatoes to cook) if you like hamburger buns on the toast grill.
2. A beef patty, a slice of tomato, onion, lettuce, and mayonnaise, or if needed, an extra slice of Parmesan cheese will be placed in each bun!

Nutrition Info

Calories: 226kcal, Calcium: 144mg, Carbohydrates: 4g, Protein: 29g, Fat: 9g, Vitamin C: 6.3mg, Saturated Fat: 4g, Cholesterol: 118mg, Sodium: 253mg, Vitamin A: 395IU, Potassium: 529mg, Sugar: 2g, Iron: 3.1mg

47. PORK BARBECUE SLOPPY JOE SANDWICHES

Total: 35 mins

Prep: 15 mins

Cook: 20 mins

Ingredients

- 1 1/2 to 2 pounds lean ground pork
- 1 tbsp vegetable oil
- 1 cup of onion
- 1/2 cup of bell pepper
- 1 clove garlic
- 1 cup of ketchup
- 1/4 cup of water
- 1 1/2 tbsp Worcestershire sauce
- 1 1/2 tbsp brown sugar
- 1 tsp black pepper
- 1/4 tsp cayenne pepper
- Dash ground allspice
- 6 to 8 buns

Steps to Make It

1. Use lean pork or smear 1 1/2 to 2 pounds of pork far or lean pork shoulder in this recipe.
2. Heat the oil in a large skillet over medium-high heat. Add pork and cook, stir and break until no pink is left. Remove a plate and set aside.
3. Add the onion and pepper, and cook, stirring, about 4 minutes until the onion is brightly browned. Add the garlic and simmer for 2 minutes. Stir in the skillet the

pork and then add the ketchup, water, Worcestershire sauce, brown sugar, peppers, and allspice. Bring to a frying pan. Simmer, uncovered, occasionally stirring for approximately 10 minutes.

4. Add salt, if necessary, and taste.
5. Serve with coleslaw and fries oversplit, toasted buns.

48. QUICK AND EASY VEGETABLE BEEF SOUP

Prep Time: 15 mins

Cook Time: 30 mins

Total Time: 45 mins

Ingredients

- 1 pound lean ground beef
- ½ chopped onion
- 2 cloves chopped garlic
- 32-ounce beef broth
- 2 medium potatoes, peeled and chopped into 3/4-inch chunks
- 8-ounce tomato sauce
- 14.5-ounce undrained petite diced tomatoes
- 16-ounce frozen mixed soup vegetables
- salt
- pepper
- 1 tbsp white vinegar

Instructions

1. Brown the ground beef over medium heat in a big pot. Drain away any excess fat.
2. Go back to the pot and add the onions. Cook for 3 minutes or so. Add garlic and cook, constantly mix, for about a minute. Add the broth of beef and potatoes sliced. Bring to boil. Bring to boil. Cook for about 5 minutes and add tomato sauce, tomatoes, and mixed frozen vegetables. Return to the boil, reduce the heat to a simmer, and cover.
3. Cook until tender potatoes and vegetables. To taste, add salt and pepper. Then add a tbsp of white vinegar before serving for an extra taste.

49. LETTUCE LEAF TACOS

Prep: 20 mins

Cook: 20 mins

Total: 40 mins

Ingredients

- 1 green chopped bell pepper
- 1 yellow chopped onion
- 2 tbsp olive oil
- 2 tbsp chicken stock
- 1 pound ground beef
- 3 tbsp taco seasoning
- 2 large Roma chopped tomatoes
- ½ tsp salt
- 8 ounce shredded Cheddar cheese
- 12 large romaine lettuce leaves

Directions

1. Cook and stir with olive oil and chicken broth, green bell pepper, and yellow onion in a skillet over medium heat until the ounce is translucent around 5 minutes.
2. 2. Break the beef into small sections. Place it over medium heat in a separate skillet. Cook and add a taco to ground beef until browned and crumbly, 5 to 8 minutes. Drain excess fat.
3. In a cup, sprinkle Roma tomatoes with salt. In a separate bowl, place the Cheddar cheese.
4. Complete each lettuce with approximately two tbsp beef; 1 to 2 tsp green pepper mixture, Roma tomato, approximately 1 1/2 tbsp of Cheddar cheese.

Nutrition Info

Per Serving:

cholesterol 127.7mg ; 550 calories; carbohydrates 14.4g ; cholesterol 127.7mg ; protein 34.5g ; cholesterol 127.7mg fat 38.9g ; sodium 1223.4mg.

50. PANKO-BREADED PORK CHOPS

Total: 20 mins

INGREDIENTS

- 1 large egg
- 1 cup of Japanese bread crumbs
- 2 tbsp freshly grated Parmesan cheese
- 1 tsp minced sage
- Salt and freshly ground pepper
- Four 3/4-inch-thick pork chops
- 1/4 cup of extra-virgin olive oil

Directions

1. Beat the egg gently in a shallow bowl. Toss the panko onto a plate with the sage, 1/2 salt tsp, and 1/8 pepper tsp. Season the pork chops with salt and pepper. Spray the chops into the egg and press into the seasoned crumbs.

ADVERTISEMENT

- Heat the olive oil in a large nonstick skillet until shimmering. Add the chops and fry for about 10 minutes, occasionally turning to brown gold and cooked. Transfer the cutlery to the plate and serve.

51. BEEF AND BUTTERNUT SQUASH STEW

Prep Time: 15 minutes

Cook Time: 3 hours

Total Time: 3 hours 15 minutes

Ingredients

- 2 pounds peeled and cubed Butternut Squash
- 3 - 4 tbsp Olive Oil
- 1 large chopped onion
- 2 pounds lean beef chuck
- 32 ounces Beef Stock
- 2 cloves crushed garlic
- sprig fresh thyme
- sprig of rosemary
- 1 tsp salt
- 1 tsp pepper

Instructions

2. Prepare squash, peel it, remove the seeds and cut into cubes.
3. If your beef is not already cut in half, cut the beef into cubes, and onion the same thing.
4. Heat the oil in a large pot at medium heat, then add the onion and sap for a couple of minutes, then add the beef and brown for a few minutes.
5. Add stock of beef, herbs, salt, and pepper.
6. Cook for about an hour with a lid on the pot on the top of the stove, do not boil.
7. Then add the squash and cook for 30 minutes, or until the beef is tender.

SLOW COOKER INSTRUCTIONS:

1. Follow the directions, saute the onions, and brown the beef.
2. Now you want to add to the slow cooker the beef, onions, butterfly squash, and all other ingredients.
3. Cook it for 5 to 6 hours or around 3 to 4 hours at low. I will check it after three hours to see if the meat is soft and the squash is soft. How long it is going to depend on the heat of your slow cooker.
4. I have two slow cookers, and in the high and low settings, the newer is cooler than, the older.

Recipe Notes

- I found it hard to find the paleo bought in the supermarket or 30 whole beef broth for this recipe, so you might need to use homemade beef broth, or you could only use water as an alternative.
- A good pan with a heavy bottom, or a Dutch oven, will be required to make this stew on the stovetop. If your pan is skinny, almost certainly, your stew will burn before it is cooked.
- Alternatively, you can easily cook it in a slow cooker that works well.

Nutrition Information

Beef and Butternut Squash Stew

Amount Per Serving

Calories 282Calories from Fat 72

Saturated Fat 3g

Fat 8g

Sodium 561mg

Cholesterol 88mg

Potassium 880mg

Carbohydrates 16g

Fibre 2g

Sugar 3g

Protein 34g

Vitamin A 12055IU2

Calcium 75mg

Vitamin C 25.1mg

Iron 3.9mg

52. LOADED RADISH CHIP NACOS

PREP TIME: 15 MINS

COOK TIME: 20 MINS

TOTAL TIME: 35 MINS

Ingredients

- 15-18 thinly sliced radishes - 2 bunches
- 1 tbsp olive oil - enough to lightly coat the radish slices
- 1/2 diced bell pepper
- 1/2 cup of rinsed and drained black beans
- 1 serrano pepper; seeded and diced; can sub jalapeno

- 3/4 cup of shredded Mexican cheese
- 1 diced avocado
- 2 tbsp chopped cilantro
- 1 lime - for serving

Instructions

1. Heat the oven to 400 degrees F. Line two parchment paper baking sheets.
2. Prepare the radishes by washing them and chopping up and down. Run through a mandolin each radish to make thin slices. If you have no mandolin, use a sharp knife to slice the radishes carefully.
3. In a mixing bowl, thrust the radish in olive oil until they are coated very thinly. Transfer to the baker and spread them overlapping open. Bake for 13-15 minutes or until crisp, shrink, and wrinkly. Check your progress from 10 minutes to make sure you don't burn.
4. During the baking process, prepare the other ingredients by dicing the bell pepper, serrano pepper, avocado, and cilantro. If the cheese isn't already shredded, Drain and rinse the black beans, shred the cheese.
5. When the radius is ready, transfer them all to a baking sheet (keep the parchment paper underneath them). Push them without overlapping to the middle. Radish chips and chopped peppers, black beans, and cheese. Top with chopped chips.
6. For another 3-4 minutes, cook the nachos or until the cheese is melted. Take them with avocado, cilantro, and a squeeze of lime juice from the oven and top them. Divide into two to three parts and pass to serving plates!

Nutrition

Serving: 1serving | Calories: 467kcal | Carbohydrates: 30g | Protein: 17g | Fat: 34g | Saturated Fat: 10g | Polyunsaturated Fat: 1g | Monounsaturated Fat: 5g | Cholesterol: 40mg | Sodium: 557mg | Potassium: 1293mg | Fiber: 15g | Sugar: 7g | Vitamin A: 1410IU | Vitamin C: 95mg | Calcium: 373mg | Iron: 3mg

53. GARLIC PARMESAN FRIES

Prep Time: 10 mins

Cook Time: 20 mins

Total Time: 30 mins

Ingredients

- oven chips (250g)
- Butter (1 tsp)
- clove garlic (2)
- ½ cup of Parmesan cheese
- ¼ cup of parsley

Instructions

1. Heat the oven and cook the oven chips as instructed by the packet.
2. I always get much better results if I use a mesh or a crisper tray for cooking chips for the oven.
3. Connect the garlic and cook in a big pot. Melt the butter over low heat release all the flavours slowly. If cooked to too high a temperature, garlic can burn easily, so keep the heat low.

4. When the oven chips are cooked and brown golden, add them to the butter and rub the chip in the garlic butter evenly.
5. Add parmesan grated and parsley (if used and stir well. Serve instantly.

Notes

- Buy high quality fried ovens because that makes a difference to the final result.
- Don't use chips! Make Parmesan garlic wedges, or even add some garlic to a roast potato to a savoury chicken.
- Vary the amount of garlic according to your preference. If you are a vegetarian, use hard cheese in the veggie grana style.
- Make your own chips. Make your own. Cook the chips as usual and in a deep-fat fryer or Actifry or another air fryer, then add to the mixture of the garlic butter. Then add the Parmesan as mentioned above.
- Make twice the amount of garlic butter for quick and hassle-free chips and freeze half it. Next time you're looking for Parmesan garlic chips, just melt the butter in a frying pan and add the chips.
- Bake them on a mesh tray for crisper oven chips. This cost just a few pounds, lasts for years, and goes through the dishwasher without any problems. You make a real difference and buy more.
- Serve Parmesan fried garlic or wedges immediately. You can heat them on a baking tile in the oven, but they are not almost as new.

Nutrition Info

Garlic Parmesan Fries

Amount Per Serving

Calories 448Calories from Fat 243

Fibre 6g

Calcium 323mg

Fat 27g

Saturated Fat 11g

Vitamin A 890IU

Cholesterol 22mg

Sodium 1036mg

Potassium 602mg

Carbohydrates 40g

Sugar 1g

Protein 13g

Vitamin C 19mg

Iron 2mg

54. CHINESE BEEF AND BROCCOLI STIR FRY RECIPE

Prep Time: 30 mins

Cook Time: 10 mins

Total Time: 40 mins

INGREDIENTS

- 1 pound beef round steak or flank steak, sliced lengthwise into 2 1/2 inch wide pieces and then crosswise into 1/8 inch thick slices. Try to freeze the beef for an hour or two to make it firm easier slicing.
- 3 tbsp + 1 tsp divided soy sauce
- 5 tsp divided brown sugar
- 4 tsp cornstarch
- 5–7 tbsp peanut oil, corn oil
- 2 tbsp rice wine sherry
- 1 tbsp hoisin sauce
- 1 tsp Chinese sesame oil
- 8 cups of bite-sized broccoli florets
- 1 tsp kosher salt
- 1/2 tsp sugar
- 4 tsp Chinese Rice Wine
- 5 tbsp water
- 1 small onion, peeled, halved, and thinly sliced
- 4 tsp finely minced ginger root
- 1 tbsp minced garlic
- 1/2 tsp crushed red pepper flakes

INSTRUCTIONS

1. *Marinate the Beef*: In a small bowl, combine whisk marinade ingredients such as soy sauce (2 tbsp), brown sugar, and peanut oil (1 tbsp). Put in a plastic bag, beef, and marinade. Massage the meat with the marinade in the bag. Click out the air, seal the bag, and marinate at room temp for 30 minutes or in the fridge for up to 24 hours. Carry to the temple of the space. Until usage until.

2. *Make the Sauce*: In a small bowl, combine rice wine or sherry (2 tbsp), brown sugar (4 tsp), soy sauce (4 tsp), hoisin sauce (1 tbsp), and sesame oil (1 tsp).

3. *Stir-Fry Broccoli*: Heat a wok (or large, heavy skillet) overheat to warm enough to evaporate a drop of water immediately. Add 2 tbsp of oil to the wok and coat with a swirl. Reduce to medium-high heat. Add broccoli, stir-fry, and constantly toss for a minute. Sprinkle broccoli with 1 salt tsp and 1/2 sugar tsp. Well, to toss, to coat. Add the wine of rice (4 tsp). Give it a nice stir after it hisses. Add water (5 tbsp) and cook the liquid. Cover the wok and leave the broccoli steam until soft but still crisp, for 3-4 minutes. Transfer the broccoli into a big bowl and clean the wok out.

4. *Stir-Fry Beef and Complete the Dish*: Return to high heat wok. Apply 2 cucharks of oil and swirl to coat. Reduce medium-high sun. Stir in the onion and fry for a minute. Add 4 tsp of ginger, garlic (1 tbsp), and 1/2 tsp of pepper to the plate. Stir fry until aromatic for about 10 seconds. Add the beef and brush actively until 90 per cent of the rosé is gone and add additional oil to avoid sticking, if necessary. Add a stir to the sauce and pour into the wok. Toss the beef with sauce to coat it. Return the broccoli to the wok and cook until all of the beef is fully

cooked and heated. Transfer the stir-fry to a large dish and serve with white rice, whenever you want.

NOTES

Make-ahead strategies:

- You can cut broccoli into florets, wrap it in a damp paper towel, stuff it in a ziplock baggy and keep it up to 24 hours in the fridge.
- The beef can be cut and marinated for up to 24 hours. Bring until use to room temperature.

55. SAVORY CHEDDAR CHEESE BISCUIT

PREP: 10 mins

BAKE: 15 to 18 mins

TOTAL: 25 mins

Ingredients

- 2 cups of King Arthur Unbleached Self-Rising Flour
- 4 ounces cheddar cheese, the sharper, the better;
- 1 cup of heavy cream

Instructions

1. Heat the oven to 425°F, with a rack in the top third.
2. Cut the cheese into a few chunks to produce the biscuits using a food processor. Place the cheese and flour into your food processor's work tank.
3. Method to smooth the mix; the cheese is very finely sliced.
4. Add the cream and pulse until the paste is cohesive. Transfer the paste to a slightly blurred surface.

56. STRAWBERRY RED ZINGER TEA JELLY

Prep time: 5 mins
Cook time: 5 mins
Total time: 10 mins

Ingredients

- 3 tsp agar agar
- 1 cup of water
- 2 Celestial Red Zinger tea bags
- 1 cup of apple juice
- 1 cup of hulled and sliced strawberries

Instructions

1. As per product instructions, prepare and dissolve gelatine or agar.
2. Preparation of gelatine: dissolve gelatine in 1 cup of boiling water and add apple juice and sugar. Steep 5 minutes of tea bags and then discard to set the refrigerate. If the jelly begins to firm, add strawberries into the jelly mixture. Agar preparation: Into a saucepan of agar powder and water, heat until dissolved (do not boil). (do not boil). (do not boil). (do not boil). (do not boil). (do not boil). Add sugar and apple juice and liquid steep tea bags for 5 minutes, then discard bags. Place in the mould the sliced strawberries and pour the liquid over the end.
3. Chill overnight, or schedule 24 hours.

57. CHOCOLATE CHIA SEED PUDDING

PREP TIME: 5 mins

WAIT TIME: 4 hrs

TOTAL TIME: 4 hrs 5 min

INGREDIENTS

- US Customary - Metric
- 2 tbsp cacao powder
- 2 tbsp maple syrup
- 1 tsp vanilla extract
- 1 cup of dairy-free milk
- 1/4 cup of chia seeds
- Garnish
- raspberries
- chocolate shavings
- coconut whipped cream
- nuts and seeds

INSTRUCTIONS

1. Add cacao powder, maple syrup, vanilla extract, dairy milk and chia seeds in a medium-size cup. Whisk together to mix both ingredients.
2. Leave the mixture in the bowl for 15 minutes without stirring to gel for the chia seeds. After fifteen minutes, whisk it again together.

3. Cover the bowl and place overnight or a minimum of 4 hours in the refrigerator.
4. Remove the chocolate chia seed pudding from the fridge and stir a spoon. Serve in tiny glasses of dessert size. Top with your favourite fruit, shavings of chocolate or other decorations.

LISA'S TIPS

- If you find that your chia seeds don't start to thicken and gel after 10 minutes, you may have dud chia seeds. This can happen in your cupboard for a while. Only take a fresh bag of seeds of chia.
- If you want to look on your berries the frosty, this is how you do it. Freeze fresh berries in one layer on a plate that is washed and fully dry. When frozen, add to the chocolate pudding. They're going to get the frosty look about 2-3 minutes later (as they come to room temperature). But serve them easily because it's not long!

NUTRITION INFORMATION

CALORIES: 232kcal, CARBOHYDRATES: 30g, PROTEIN: 8g, FAT: 9g, SATURATED FAT: 1g, SODIUM: 65mg, POTASSIUM: 380mg, FIBER: 10g, SUGAR: 15g, VITAMIN A: 465iu, VITAMIN C: 10.6mg, CALCIUM: 328mg, IRON: 3mg

58. BANANA PROTEIN SHAKE

Prep Time: 2 mins

Cook Time: 2 mins

Total Tim: 4 mins

Ingredients

- 1 cup of plain unsweetened almond milk
- 1/2 cup of plain Greek fat yoghurt
- 1 vanilla scoop protein powder
- 1 banana frozen.
- ground cinnamon (1/8 tsp)
- ice as needed

Instructions

1. Through the blender, incorporate the unsweetened almond milk, fat grey yoghurt, vanilla protein powder, frozen bananas, and ground cinnamon.
2. Mix until it's smooth.
3. If your shake is too thick, you should add some more milk gradually to the blender.

Recipe Notes

- I recommend it because it will make the texture of the shake more creamy and thicker and so that you don't have to use much if any additional ice that can dilute the flavour. I like to freeze bananas in advance with reusable silicone bags which are perfect for storing food. That's all I use.
- You can substitute any frozen fruit of your choice if you want to enjoy this protein shake, but you don't care for

the banana or are allergic. Such great choices include cherries, strawberries, blackberries, avocado, pineapple, mangoes, raspberries or a mix.

- If you're not vegan, you can also quickly omit the Greek yoghurt. Although the texture contributes useful nutrients and creaminess, it can easily be made without it or with a vegan alternative, such as coconut yoghurt or other vegetable yoghurts.

Nutrition Facts

Banana Protein Shake

Amount Per Serving (1 protein shake)

Calories 362Calories from Fat 96

Fat 10.7g

Saturated Fat 0.1g

Cholesterol 19.2mg

Sodium 208.8mg

Carbohydrates 32.6g

Fibre 6g

Sugar 19.2g

Protein 38.2g

59. VANILLA PROTEIN SHAKE

Prep Time: 5 minutes

Total Time: 5 minutes

INGREDIENTS

- 1 ½ cups of cashew milk
- 1–2 dates
- 1 tbsp raw cashews
- ½ tsp vanilla bean
- 1 serving Protein Smoothie Boost

INSTRUCTIONS

1. In a mixer, combine all ingredients.
2. Pour into a glass and instantly enjoy. Feel free to add ice to refresh it.

NOTES

- You can use other plant protein powder if your preference varies, but the taste, sweetness and nutrients differ.

NUTRITION INFO

Serving Size: 1 smoothie

Sugar: 32.5g, Fiber: 11.3g, Calories: 347, Carbohydrates: 48.4g, Sodium: 298.8mg, Fat: 12.7g, Protein: 15g

60. LEMON PIE PROTEIN SHAKE

Prep Time: 10 minutes

Total Time: 10 minutes

Ingredients

- 1 cup of cashew milk
- 1 cup of frozen banana slices
- 2 tbsp plant-based vanilla protein powder
- 1 tsp lemon zest
- 2 tsp lemon juice
- 1/4 tsp vanilla extract
- 1/8 tsp lemon extract
- coconut whipped cream optional
- cookie crust crumbs optional

Instructions

1. Add cashew milk or almond milk, frozen banana, protein powder, lemon zest and lemon juice to the mixer and blend until smooth. Mix.
2. Send the cream and cookie or crust pie to a glass and top, if desired.

Recipe Notes

- Make sure that your lemons remove pesticides. Fill a big bowl with 4 pieces of water into 1 slice of simple white vinegar to do so. Soak the lemons with other vegetables or fruit for 20 minutes in the mixture. Rinse well with water the fruit or vegetables.
- I suggest that you make your own cream with whipped coconut for complete control of all ingredients. Using this

basic recipe. Swerve can be used for a sugar-free version! Native Forest is a powerful brand. "Native Forest."

61. SPLIT PEA SOUP

Ready in: 2 hours

Prep: 15 minutes

Cook: 1 hour 45 minutes

Ingredients

- 1 Tbsp olive oil
- 1 1/2 cups of chopped yellow onion
- 1 1/4 cups of chopped celery
- 1 tsp minced garlic
- 4 cups of unsalted chicken broth
- 4 cups of water
- 16 ounces picked over and rinsed dried split peas
- Two bay leaves
- 1 1/2 tsp chopped fresh thyme
- Salt and freshly ground black pepper
- 1 1/2 pounds meaty ham bone shanks
- 1 cup of chopped carrots
- Chopped fresh parsley for garnish

Instructions

1. 1. Heat olive oil with medium-high heat in a large pot. Add onion and celery and saute for 3 minutes. Add 1 minute longer garlic and saute.
2. Pour in the broth and water of the chicken. Add split peas, thyme and bay leave. Add salt and pepper to taste mild (I like to wait to add more salt until the end to see how salty the ham has made the soup).

3. Nestle bone ham into a mixture of both. Bring the blend to a boil, and then decrease to low. Cover and let cook, stirring periodically, about 60 to 80 minutes until peas and ham are tender.
4. Remove soup from ham, give 10 minutes to rest, and then chop or dice portion of meat, cover.
5. Add carrots* to the soup in the meantime. Cover the soup and occasionally stir until the peas have broken down, about 30 minutes longer **. Stir occasionally.
6. Drop ham into soup, season as appropriate with more salt. Serve warm, and parsley garnished if needed.

Notes

- If needed, you can add a few yellow or red potatoes to make the carrot even hotter by adding a soup.
- When you find the soup doesn't get as thick as you want during cooking, you can let it cook for the last 30 minutes uncovered.
- Note that the soup is thickened as it slightly rests and cools. It can be diluted with more water if required.

Nutrition Info

Split Pea Soup

Amount Per Serving

Sodium 202.27mg, Calories 450g, Fat 7.64g, Saturated Fat 1.8g, Calcium 93.16mg, Cholesterol 66.67mg, Potassium 1358.31mg, Vitamin C 7.19mg, Carbohydrates 54.24g, Fiber 20.96g, Sugar 9.35g, Protein 43.24g, Vitamin A 3794.82IU, Iron 4.83mg

62. BANANA CREAM PUDDING PARFAIT

Total: 4 hrs 40 mins

Ingredients
Banana Pudding

- 1 ½ cups of divided reduced-fat milk plus 2 tbsp
- Two eaches large or three small very ripe sliced bananas
- One envelope of unflavored gelatin
- ½ cup of sugar
- ½ cup of nonfat dry milk
- ⅛ tsp kosher salt
- ½ cup of heavy cream
- ½ cup of reduced-fat plain Greek yogurt
- 1 ½ tsp vanilla extract

Layers & Topping

- Three eaches medium sliced firm-ripe bananas
- ¾ cup of coarsely chopped toasted hazelnuts

Directions

1. Prepare pudding: Place 1 1/2 cups of milk and bananas in a small non-reactive cup, and remove from heat. Cover and allow 1 hour to stand. Or cool to room temperature, cover, and cool before one day. Cool.
2. Mix the gelatin in a medium bowl with the remaining 2 tbsp of milk. Set a thin sheet over the bowl
3. In the banana-milk mixture, add sugar, dry milk, and salt; cook, stir, until the dry ingredients are dissolved, steam and milk are hot (don't leave to boil).

4. Pour the milk mixture into the gelatin through the sieve, press the bananas to remove as much milk as possible without directly cutting the pulp through the sieve. Whisk to dissolve the gelatine. (Use remaining pulp in a smoothie or muffin batter, or discard.) Cover and refrigerate for at least 3 hours and up to 5 days until firm and cold.

5. Scrape the chilled pudding into a stand mixer's bowl with a medium-high whisk and whip. First, it will look like cottage cheese, but it will continue to beat around 1 minute smoothly. Return the pudding to its jar. In a bowl, mix milk, yogurt, and vanilla and beat for five full minutes at medium-high. Fold the pudding.

6. Assemble perfect: 1/4 cup spoon pudding in each of 6 perfect bottles. Cover with 3 or 4 slices of banana and 1 1/2 table cubes of hazelnuts, and another layer of banana slices. Spoon the rest of the banana slices and hazelnuts on another 1/4 cup pudding and top. There was a mistake (To learn how to "brulee" the banana slices for the topping, see Tips.)

Tips

- Make-Ahead Tip: Prepare up to 5 days ahead by Phase 5. Finish phase 6 and cool the assembled perfects for up to 4 hours.

- When cooking with acidic foods (citrus, berries, or tomatoes), use non-reactive bowls or pots—stainless steel, enamel-coated, non-stick, or glass avoid food from interacting with the dish. Colors and/or flavors may be imparted from reactive cookware, aluminum, and cast-iron.

- Burned banana slices—sliced banana with caramelized sugar—make our banana pudding great for hardly any extra calories. You'll need a small kitchen torch to make them. Sprinkle 1/2 tsp with a slice of banana. Granulated sugar. Granulated sugar. Keep the flames 1 to 2 centimeters apart, heat, and brown the sugar. Let stand tight and cool.

Nutrition Information

Per Serving:

348 calories; protein 9.6g ; thiamin 0.2mg ; carbohydrates 40.6g ; dietary fiber 3g ; sodium 99.9mg ; sugars 32.3g; fat 18g ; potassium 517.5mg ; saturated fat 6.4g ; iron 0.9mg ; cholesterol 34.6mg ; vitamin a iu 595.8IU ; vitamin c 6.8mg ; folate 35.5mcg ; calcium 189.4mg ; magnesium 55.1mg ; added sugar 17g.

63. PEANUT PEANUT BUTTER PROTEIN SHAKE

PREP TIME10 mins

TOTAL TIME10 mins

INGREDIENTS

- 1 1/2 cups of unsweetened almond milk
- One large frozen bananas
- 1/4 cup of peanut butter
- 1-2 scoops of protein powder peptides
- 1/4 tsp pure vanilla extract
- 1 cup of crushed ice
- 1-2 handfuls fresh baby spinach optional
- Honey to taste

INSTRUCTIONS

1. In a blender, mix all the ingredients and process them smoothly. Serve instantly.

NUTRITION INFO

Iron: 2.4mg, Calories: 371kcal, Vitamin C: 13.9mg, Carbohydrates: 32g, Protein: 22g, Vitamin C: 13.9mg, Fat: 19g, Saturated Fat: 3g, Cholesterol: 6mg, Sodium: 292mg, Potassium: 960mg, Fiber: 4g, Sugar: 20g, Vitamin A: 2195IU, Calcium: 328mg

64. LOW CARB CHEESEBURGER BREAKFAST SCRAMBLE

Prep Time: 5 minutes

Cook Time: 15 minutes

Total Time: 20 minutes

INGREDIENTS

- 1 pound Ground Beef
- 6 Medium Egg
- 6 Ounces Cream Cheese
- Yellow Onion (4 Tbsps)
- Water (2 Tbsps)
- Salt & Pepper as need

INSTRUCTIONS

2. Heat the oven to 350 degrees F. Cook the ground beef in a skillet until it's no longer pink for your meat.
3. Add onion next and cook at medium-low until translucent.

4. Add the cream cheese and keep cooking until the cream cheese melts.
5. Beat the eggs and pour over the meat mixture, then add to the baker and add 5-10 minutes into the oven or until they are baked. Stir in salt and pepper. Serve warm Serve. Enjoy!

Nutrition Info

Amount Per Serving (1 Serving)

Protein 21g, Calories 430g, Carbohydrates 3g, Fat 40g

65. SWEET AND SPICY TOFU BURGERS

Prep Time: 5 mins

Cook Time: 15 mins

Total Time: 20 minutes

Ingredients

1 – 14 ounces package extra firm tofu**Marinade**

2 Tbsp tamari sauce

1 Tbsp sesame oil

1 Tbsp sriracha

1/2 Tbsp maple syrup

Spicy Mayo Sauce

1/4 cup of veganaise

1 Tbsp sriracha

1/2 Tbsp lemon juice

Instructions

1. In a large ziplock bag, mix marinade ingredients. Shake to combine. Shake to combine.
2. Drain tofu and push to drain the greatest possible excess water. Slice the tofu block to half the thickness, then use a "patties" round cookie cutter.
3. Place the tofu patties in the bag carefully and rotate several times to coat with the marinade. Cool for 30 to 4 hours to marinate.
4. In the meantime, in a small bowl, mix spicy mayo ingredients and whisk them together.
5. 5. Heat the grill and carefully arrange the grill. Grill for ten to twelve minutes on each side. Add tofu patty to a bun, pile on tops, and enjoy!

Notes

- • These can also be made in the oven! Heat the oven to 400 degrees F. Line the parchment baking and add patties on the sheet. Bake for 8-10 minutes, flip back to the oven for 8-10 more minutes.

Nutrition Information

Serving Size: 1, Unsaturated Fat: 10 g, Calories: 236, Protein: 12 g, Sugar: 6 g, Sodium: 296 mg,

Fat:12g, Saturated Fat: 2 g, Trans Fat: 0 g, Carbohydrates: 15 g, Fiber: 3 g, Cholesterol: 0 mg

66. CANNING CRUSHED OR DICED TOMATOES

Prep Time: 1 hr

Cook Time: 45 mins

Total Time: 1 hr 45 mins

Ingredients

- 15 pounds tomatoes
- bottled lemon juice

Instructions
Prepare the canning equipment:

1. Prepare your jars and your lids by washing and well rinsing in wet, soapy water. Place the jar rack into the water bath canner, place the clean jars inside the canner, add water, and sterilize the jar for 10 minutes.
2. Heat your lids over low heat in a small bath. Maintain warm jars and lids until ready to use.

Prepare the tomatoes:

1. Clean in clear water your tomatoes.
2. Bring a big saucepan of water to a boil to peel the tomatoes, and fill a huge ice water bowl. Sprinkle the tomatoes in the boiling water and remove the skins – 30-60 seconds. Remove the tomatoes from the pot and cool down in the ice bowl. Remove water.
3. Peel your tomatoes as soon as they're cool enough. Core and trim any areas that are missing or discolored. Split into quarters or dice.

4. In a large pot, put diced tomatoes and juice and bring to a boil over medium-high heat—five minutes of cooking time. Shrink to low heat and stay warm.
5. Add about 1 pound (2 cups) of the quartered tomatoes to a large cup of crushed tomatoes. Simmer on low heat for about 5 minutes before tomatoes soften and release their fluid. Crush with a potato master softly. Increase the heat to medium and boil the tomato juice. Mix often to avoid sticking.
6. When the tomatoes boil, add the remaining quartered tomatoes and stir for 5 minutes. They don't have to crush; they will soften as they cook. Reduce heat to low and retain warmth.

Can the diced or crushed tomatoes:

1. Spread a towel on the counter. Spread. Using your jar lifter to remove warm jars from the towel and drain them. Add 1/4 tsp of citric acid to each jar or 1 tbsp of bottled lemon juice.
2. Use the funnel and ladle, fill the warm jars with hot tomatoes, leaving a headspace of 1/2 inch. Using your popper to stir up air bubbles in the jars. Remove the rims. Use your magnetic lift to lift the lid out of the warm water, center the jar lid and screw it onto the strip until it's secure.
3. Place jars in canner with a jar lifter, leaving space between them. When all jars are in the canner, the water level is balanced so that it is at least one pound above the top of the jar. If required, add more hot water so that the water level is one inch above the jar's top. Pour the water between the jars and not directly on them when applied. Using the hot water in the little pot that your lids have been in.

4. Cover the canner and bring high heat to a boil. Once the water boils vigorously, it pints at altitudes below 1000 feet for 35 minutes (adjust processing time for your height if necessary).
5. When the processing time is done, turn off the heat and cool the canner for around 10 minutes. Spread on the counter a kitchen towel; tilt off the cover so that the steam will not burn your skin. You are using a jar lift to carefully lift jars from the canner and place them on the towel. Cool the jars for 12 to 24 hours. The acceptable ping of the jar lids should be heard.
6. After 12 to 24 hours, make sure that the jar lids are closed by pressing the lid's middle. The cover is not meant to pop up. If the body bends up and down, it doesn't stick. Cool the jar and use it in a few days.
7. Remove the belt screw and wash the jars. Mark the jars and date them. Keep your jars cool, dark, and use them within 12 months. Returns about 9-pint jars of tomatoes crushed or diced.

Recipe Notes

- This is a checked healthy canning recipe from the USDA Home Canning Guide. Changing the recipe will make the canning product unsafe.
- All times are less than 1,000 ft above sea level. Altitudes above 1,000 ft must be modified.

67. KETO OVERNIGHT OATS

Prep Time: 5 mins

Chill in the fridge: 4 hrs 5 mins

Ingredients

- 1 tbsp chia seeds
- 2 tbsp hemp seeds
- 1 tbsp coconut flour
- 1/4 cup of unsweetened shredded coconut
- 1/3 cup of unsweetened almond milk
- 1/2 tsp vanilla extract
- 2-3 tsp Monk fruit sweetener optional to taste

OPTIONAL TOPPINGS:

- berries
- toasted coconut
- sunflower seed butter
- hemp seeds

Instructions

1. In a large container or jar with the lid, add all the ingredients. Remove until combined. Cover with lid and chill for at least 4 hours in the fridge.
2. When ready to eat, remove the cover and blend until the desired consistency is achieved. Add more milk.
3. Divide between two bowls, add toppings/mix-ins, and taste.

Nutrition Information

Amount Per Serving (1 serving)

Calories 216Calories from Fat 153, Carbohydrates 9g, Protein 8g, Fat 17g, Fiber 6g, Sugar 1g

68. AVOCADO MAYO

Total Time: 5 minutes

Ingredients

- 2/3 cup of mashed ripe avocado
- 2 tsp white vinegar
- 2 tsp lemon juice
- 3/4 tsp onion powder
- 1/8 tsp garlic powder
- 1/4 tsp salt
- 1/4 cup of water
- 2 tbsp oil, for a low-fat mayo

Instructions

1. Mix all ingredients in a blender until they are smooth. Add additional water if you want a slimmer mayo spread. Please add a hot sauce or a cayenne dash if you want a spicy mayo. Store in the refrigerator for the remaining 3-4 days.

   ### Notes

- Try this Mousse Avocado Chocolate, too.

69. SAVORY BEEF BONE BROTH

Prep Time: 20 mins

Cook Time: 1 d 1 hr

Total Time: 1 d 1 hrs 20 mins

Ingredients

- 3-4 pounds of mixed beef bones
- 2 medium carrots coarsely chopped
- 3 celery stalks coarsely chopped
- 2 medium coarsely chopped onions
- olive oil (1 tbsp)
- apple cider vinegar (2 tbsp)
- 1 bay leaf

Instructions

1.Heat the oven to 400 degrees F. and place mixed beef bones on a roasting pan in a single layer coat evenly with olive oil.
1. Roast for 30 minutes for the bones, then roast for another 30 minutes.
2. Into a big crockpot or soup pot, bring the roasted bones, vegetables, bay leaf, and vinegar.
3. Cover entirely with water and simmer high.
4. Reduce heat to low and cook for 12-24 hours. Add water to keep all the ingredients intact.
5. When brown is black, remove the bones, vegetables, and bay leaves from the heat and spread them through a wire strainer or cheesecloth.

6. 6. Cool to room temperature. Pour into jars and let cool for at least 1 hour in the refrigerator.
7. Heat to the appropriate temperature when you are ready to serve.

Notes

- Since they are strained out, marginal carbs are added from the vegetables. You can leave carrots away and add more celery if desired. You should add herbs and seasonings to your taste.

Nutrition

Carbohydrates: 1g | Calories: 69 | Fiber: 0g | Protein: 6g | Fat: 4g

70. SIMPLE STRAWBERRY SMOOTHIE RECIPE

prep time: 5 MINUTES

total time: 5 MINUTES

Ingredients

- 3 cups frozen strawberries
- 1 1/2 cups of any variety of milk
- 1/3 cup of strawberry jam

Instructions

1. In a blender, place the frozen strawberries, backup, and milk.
2. Place the lid above the end.
3. Puree to smooth.

Notes

- Mix it up! Try the preserve of blackberry and frozen blackberries with frozen bits of mango or mango jelly.

Nutrition Info

serving: 8ounces, calcium: 126mg, calories: 169kcal, carbohydrates: 32g, vitamin c: 66mg, protein: 3g, fat: 3g, saturated fat: 1g, fiber: 2g, cholesterol: 9mg, vitamin a: 160iu, sodium: 49mg, potassium: 307mg, sugar: 23g, iron: 0.6mg

71. BUTTERNUT SQUASH PURE

PREP TIME: 10 mins

COOK TIME: 45 mins

TOTAL TIME: 55 mins

Ingredients

- 2 whole halved and seeded butternut squash
- 6 tbsp. butter, cut into pieces
- 1/4 cup of pure maple syrup
- Dash Of salt
- The ground cinnamon, for sprinkling

Directions

1. Heat the oven to 375 degrees F. Place the squash half, cut down the side, fried, and roast for 30-40 minutes, or fork.
2. Scoop out the innards and add butter, syrup, and salt to the dish. Pump with a potato masher OR a food processor puree.
3. Sprinkle with cinnamon and spread into a small casserole dish. Keep warm in the oven, then serve with a spoonful!

72. BROCCOLI CHEDDAR SOUP RECIPE

Prep time: 15 minutes

Cook time: 30 minutes

INGREDIENTS

- 1 large head or two small heads of broccoli, chopped into florets and stems
- 1/4 cup of unsalted butter
- 1/2 white chopped onion
- 1 small peeled and grated carrot
- 1/4 cup of all-purpose flour
- 1-quart vegetable stock
- 2 cups of whole milk
- 8 ounces grated cheddar cheese
- 1 tsp salt
- 1/8 tsp fresh black pepper
- Bread, for serving

METHOD

1 Blanch the broccoli: Carry a big pot of water to a boil and add a few big salt pinches. Add broccoli stalks and blanch for 2 - 3 minutes until bright green and slightly crispy, yet tender fork.

Broccoli drain. Draw off and reserve around 1 cup of the florets.

Broccoli Cheddar Soup Broccoli Blanch

2 Cook the onions and carrots: Wipe the pot out, bring it to medium heat, and melt the butter. When melting, add the onions and carrots and cook, continually stirring, until veggies are tender, 4 to 5 minutes.

Broccoli Cheddar Soup Broccoli Broccoli Cheddar Soup Fried Onions and Carrots Broccoli Soup

3 Cook the soup: Remove all-purpose meal. The meal is a paste with the vegetables. Cook the vegetables for a minute or two, then slowly pour them into the vegetable stock. Continuously stir as you pour into the store to prevent lumps.

After adding all of the stock, bring the soup to a low frying glass. Add milk and blanched broccoli (except for topping savings). Simmer for about 10 minutes over the low sun.

Sup Boil the Soup Broccoli Cheddar

4 Puree the soup: Mix with an immersion blender or allow the soup to cool until it stops steaming and batches in the mixer. (When using a mixer, make sure the soup gets cool and don't overfill the mixer to prevent spreading hot soup!)

5 Season to taste and serve: Add the rubbed cheese, salt, and pepper to the soup and blend in low heat until the cheese is melted. Sample the soup and add salt and pepper to your liking.

In a bowl, add the soup and garnish with some reserved broccoli and extra cheese. Serve with broth.

73. DILL VEGETABLE DIP RECIPE

Prep Time: 7 minutes

Total Time: 7 minutes

Ingredients

- 1 cup of Best Foods Mayonnaise
- 1 cup of sour cream
- 1 tbsp dried parsley
- 1 1/2 tbsp dried dill weed
- 1/2 tbsp onion powder
- Salt (1/2 tsp)
- Worcestershire Sauce (2 tsp)
- lemon juice (2 tsp)
- Any pepper sprinkles

Instructions

1. Mix all ingredients and cool.
2. Serve with a vegetable platter.

Nutrition Facts

Dill Vegetable Dip Recipe

Amount Per Serving

Calories 84Calories from Fat 81

Fat 9g

Saturated Fat 2g

Cholesterol 9mg

Sodium 121mg

Potassium 28mg

Carbohydrates 1g

Fiber 1g

Sugar 1g

Protein 1g

Vitamin A 77IU

Vitamin C 1mg

Calcium 17mg

Iron 1mg

74. CHEESY CAULIFLOWER TOTS

Total time: 50 minutes

Ingredients

- **Cauliflower** – Approximately 1 entire head riced.
- **Cheese** – Shredded cheddar and mozzarella, something that melts well and goes mellow.
- **Garlic** – Use as much.
- **Spices** – Seasoning in Italy is what we need today.
- **Eggs** – For this recipe, we need 4 whole eggs. They are crucial to uniting our whole recipe.
- **Seasoning** – Salt and pepper.

How To Make Cheesy Cauliflower Tots

Heat your oven: To 425 degrees F. Prepare large baking with paper parchment.

Rice the cauliflower: Chop the cauliflower into small florets and add them to the food processor. Pulse until the cauliflower is like rice a few times.

Prepare the cauliflower: In a microwavable container, place the cooler and cover with the lid. Microwave 10 minutes. 10 minutes. In a wide bowl, position the microwave cooler and allow it to cool for approximately 5 minutes.

Combine the tossed to the cauliflower cheeses, garlic, Italian seasoning, eggs, salt, and pepper and blend until it is well blended. Take a tbsp of the cauliflower mixture, turn it into small tots, and place it on the prepared baking sheet. Echo the rest of the cauliflower.

Bake the tots: Bake until golden brown for about 30 minutes. I normally put them under the broiler for a few minutes to get the beautiful golden color.

Finish the dish: Serve with sauce pizza, sour cream, ketchup, or ranch dip.

75. VERMONT CHEDDAR MASHED POTATOES

TIME: 45 minutes

INGREDIENTS

- 3 pounds medium peeled and quartered russet potatoes
- ¾ pound grated Vermont aged white Cheddar
- ½ tsp baking powder
- 1 tsp kosher salt
- Black pepper, as need
- Small pinch cayenne
- Pinch of grated nutmeg
- 6 tbsp melted unsalted butter
- ¾ cup of heated heavy cream
- 2 lightly beaten eggs

PREPARATION

1. Boil potatoes in well-salted water for about 15 minutes until tender. Drain well in the colander and place the wire whisk in the bowl of a stand mixer. Beat 2 to 3 minutes at medium speed to allow the steam to escape.
2. 2. Stir in cheese, baking, salt, pepper, cayenne, and nutmeg. Beat for a minute or so again.
3. Add butter and cream, slowly blend, then raise to medium speed and sprinkle with the beaten eggs. Stop and scrape the bowl with the rubber spatula to ensure that the ingredients are uniformly integrated. Beat at medium-high intensity, 2-3 minutes, until the mixture is smooth.

4. Serve immediately in a hot bowl. Alternatively, transfer potatoes to the baking of 2 thirds, cover with paper and allow to stand at room temperature. Reheat at 350 degrees for 30 to 40 minutes, until piping is hot. (When you want the top to be browned, remove the foil halfway through the baking process.)

76. KETO VANILLA FROZEN YOGURT

Prep Time: 5 minutes

Cook Time: 0 minutes

Freezing: 30 minutes

Total Time: 35 minutes

Ingredients

- ½ cup of Greek Yoghurt full fat
- 3 tbsp Heavy Cream
- 4 tsp Sukrin Melis or your preferred powdered sweetener
- 1 tsp Vanilla Essence

Instructions

1. In a small mixing bowl, place all ingredients and combine well.
2. Glue in a ziplock bag until the mixture is uniformly distributed.
3. Freeze until the mixture is partly frozen for 20-30 minutes.
4. Cut out the corner and squeeze the mixture into 2 plates.
5. Enjoy it or enjoy your favorite toppings.

Nutrition

Calories: 126kcal | Carbohydrates: 2.5g | Protein: 6g | Fat: 9g | Saturated Fat: 6g | Cholesterol: 34mg | Sodium: 32mg | Sugar: 2g | Vitamin A: 364IU | Calcium: 81mg

77. MIXED BERRY CRUMBLE CAKE

Prep Time: 15 mins

Cook Time: 42 mins

Total Time: 57 mins

Ingredients

- Crumble Topping:
- 3/4 cups of rolled oats
- 1/2 cup of all-purpose flour
- 1/4 cup of packed light brown sugar
- 1/4 cup of chopped pecans
- ¼ tsp salt
- 1/2 cup of 1/2 stick cold unsalted butter, cut into cubes
- Cake:
- ¼ cup + 2 tbsp softened unsalted butter, add more for the dish
- 1 1/2 cups of all-purpose flour add more for the dish
- 3/4 cups of granulated sugar
- 2 large eggs
- 1/2 tbsp baking powder
- ¼ tsp salt
- 1/2 cup of whole milk

- 1/2 tbsp vanilla extract
- 1 cup of fresh blueberries
- 1 cup of fresh raspberries

Instructions

1. Mix the oats, flour, brown sugar, pecan, and salt in a medium bowl first. Add butter and knead until the mixture looks rough.
2. Then make a cake, heat it to a temperature of 350 degrees F. Lightly butter baking of 8x8 inch. Dust with extra flour and tap out. Beat butter on medium to smooth for around 2 minutes with an electric mixer. Add granulated sugar and beat for about 3 minutes until light and fluffy. Add the eggs and beat them one by one. In a bowl, whisk bakery powder, salt, and meal. With a low-flour mixer, add a meal in 3 additions to the butter mixture, alternate with milk, start and end with flour, toss well after each addition. Beat in vanilla. Beat in vanilla—shift batter to the baking.
3. Mix in a big bowl the blueberries, raspberries, and half the rounding; sprinkle the mixture with the batter. Top the majority of the crumble.
4. Bake until the toothpick in the middle of the cake comes out clean, cool, and sprinkle with powdered sugar 42 minutes before serving.

78. NEAPOLITAN SMOOTHIE

READY IN: 5mins

INGREDIENTS

- Two bananas
- 1 cup of milk
- 1 cup of vanilla yogurt
- 2 tbsp cocoa
- 2 cups of strawberries
- 2 tsp vanilla
- 2 tbsp sugar

DIRECTIONS

1. Combine all ingredients in a mixer.
2. Combine and enjoy!

79. EGG WHITE AND SPINACH PIZZA

Prep Time: 5 mins

Cook Time: 5 mins

Total Time: 10 mins

Ingredients

- 1/2 cup of egg whites
- 2 tbsp. marinara sauce
- shredded mozzarella cheese (2 tbsp.)
- A splash of seasoning in Italy

- Garlic powder dash
- Small handful fresh chopped spinach
- Salt and pepper as need

Instructions

1. In a small bowl, mix egg whites.
2. Sprinkle an 8-inch pan over medium heat. Coat the spray with the kitchen (or coconut oil or butter) and place in the pan with the egg whites.
3. Push the egg edges gently into the middle of the pot and let the uncooked eggs roll out to the outside of the pot (see the video to see the demo).
4. Add salt, pepper, Italian seasoning, and garlic powder to the eggs. If the eggs are set and fried, add tomato sauce, cheese, and spinach. Place the lid over the egg pizza and cook until the cheese melts or for another minute.
5. Run out of the pan and enjoy!

Nutrition

Calories: 159kcal | Carbohydrates: 3g | Protein: 20g | Fat: 7g | Saturated Fat: 4g | Cholesterol: 23mg | Sodium: 542mg | Potassium: 296mg | Fiber: 1g | Sugar: 2g | Vitamin A: 330IU | Vitamin C: 2.1mg | Calcium: 149mg | Iron: 0.3mg

80. ANTIPASTO PASTA SALAD

PREP TIME: 20 minutes

COOK TIME: 10 minutes

TOTAL TIME: 30 minutes

Ingredients

- 8 ounces rotini pasta
- 1-pint cherry tomatoes halved
- 6 ounces jar marinated artichoke hearts quartered & drained
- ⅓ cup of sliced red onion
- ½ cup of black olives green
- 4 ounces sliced salami halved
- 8 ounces bocconcini
- 2 tbsp fresh basil sliced
- 1 tbsp fresh parsley

Dressing

- 1 cup of bottled Italian dressing
- ¼ cup of red wine vinegar
- ⅓ cup of olive oil
- ½ tsp garlic powder
- ½ tsp dried basil
- salt & pepper to taste

Instructions

1. Cook pasta al dente as instructed in the box. Rinse well and drain well under cold water.

2. Combine all dressing ingredients in a bowl and combine the whisk.
3. In a large bowl, throw all ingredients and cool them at least 1 hour before serving.

Recipe Notes

- Nutritional data are calculated using home-made dressing.

NUTRITION INFORMATION

Calories: 486, Carbohydrates: 35g, Protein: 17g, Fat: 31g, Saturated Fat: 7g, Cholesterol: 29mg, Sodium: 750mg, Potassium: 341mg, Fiber: 3g, Sugar: 4g, Vitamin A: 805IU, Vitamin C: 25.5mg, Calcium: 169mg, Iron: 1.8mg

81. VEGAN CREAMY GARLIC PASTA SAUCE

Prep time: 8 mins

Cook time: 2 mins

Total time: 10 mins

Ingredients

- Pasta of choice, cooked & 1 cup of liquid reserved
- 1-2 tsp garlic seasoning
- 1 -1½ cups of unsweetened plant-based milk of choice
- ½ cup of raw cashews, soaked overnight
- 1 tbsp olive oil
- lemon juice (1-2 tbsp)
- nutritional yeast (1 tbsp)
- onion powder (1 tsp)
- sea salt (½ tsp)
- Pepper and Red Pepper Flakes, as need

Instructions

1. Cook pasta of choice.
2. Mix garlic, cashews, plant milk, olive oil, lemon juice, nutritional yeast, and onion powder in a blender. Blend until creamy and smooth.
3. Drain pasta, leave a minimum of 1 cup of liquid cooking.
4. Return pasta to the pot, add veggie supplements, and top with sauce pasta creamy garlic. To start with, add a 1/4 cup of pasta water. Give it all a toss over medium heat and add more pasta water to make a silky sauce as required. Add salt, pepper, and spice to taste and add as needed.
5. Serve and decorate

6. The sauce is kept in the fridge for 3-5 days. It is thicker, simply thin with reserved pasta sauce or vegetable broth when used on pasta-free vegetables.

Nutrition Information

Serving size: ¼ cup of Fat: 5.7g Carbohydrates: 2.8g, Fiber: 0.8g Sugar: 0.6g, Protein: 2.9g, sauce Calories: 74

82. VEGAN CINNAMON APPLE PIE SMOOTHIE

Prep Time: 5 minutes

Total Time: 5 minutes

Ingredients

- • 1 1/2 to 2 ripe, peeled, cut and frozen bananas1 apple, peeled, seeded, and quartered
- 1 cup of vanilla almond milk
- 1 tbsp almond butter
- 1/2 tsp ground cinnamon
- pinch of ground nutmeg

Topping Ideas

- chia seeds
- ground cinnamon
- walnuts
- apple pieces
- almond butter

Instructions

1. In a strong blender, add the frozen bananas, apple, almond milk, almond butter, cinnamon, and nutmeg.
2. Mix well for 1-2 minutes or until creamy and smooth.
3. Fill in a bottle, add tapestries, and serve.

83. AVOCADO SALAD RECIPE

Prep Time: 20 minutes

Total Time: 20 minutes

Ingredients

- 3 avocados
- 3 limes
- 9 ounces mozzarella cheese
- 1/2 cup of cilantro leaves from about 10 sprigs chopped
- 2 cups of cherry tomatoes
- 1/2 red onion
- extra-virgin olive oil (3 tbsp.)
- 1/2 tsp. salt + to taste
- 1/2 tsp. black pepper + to taste
- Apple cider vinegar lime juice. (2 tbsp.)
- Instructions

Prep the Onion

1. Slicing the red onion thinly.
2. Soak the onion for 15 minutes in cold water to remove the onion sharpness.

Prep the Avocado

1. Slice the avocado halfway down the length and remove the pit.
2. Keep half of the avocado in your hand's palm. Cut the avocado in 3/8" strips without cutting through the peel diagonally.
3. Then diagonally slice the avocado without removing the peel.
4. Using a tea cubicle to pick the cut avocado out into a small bowl.
5. Press the lime juice over the avocado and set aside.

Prep The Ingredients

1. Cut the cheese into around 3/8" cubes.
2. Remove and chop the cilantro leaves. You want approximately 1/2 cup of cilantro loosely packed.
3. Half the cherry tomatoes.

Assemble the Salad

1. Add all the ingredients to your mixing bowl and mix them very gently.
2. Serve instantly.

Notes

- This salad is not well kept. Serve instantly at room temperature.

Substitutions:

- The following are delicious salad combinations.
- Queso fresco or mozzarella panela cheese.
- Chopped cherry tomatoes or standard cherry tomatoes.
- Red onion white onion.

Nutrition

Calories: 567kcal | Carbohydrates: 24g | Protein: 18g | Fat: 48g | Saturated Fat: 13g | Cholesterol: 50mg | Sodium: 660mg | Potassium: 1024mg | Fiber: 12g | Sugar: 5g | Vitamin A: 1176IU | Vitamin C: 48mg | Calcium: 371mg | Iron: 2mg

84. CINNAMON ROLL OVERNIGHT OATS

Active: 5 mins

Total: 8 hrs

Ingredients

- 2 ½ cups of 2 1/2 cups of old-fashioned rolled oats
- 2 ½ cups of 2 1/2 cups of unsweetened non-dairy milk, such as almond
- 8 tsp light brown sugar
- 2 ½ tsp vanilla extract
- 1 ¼ tsp ground cinnamon
- ½ tsp salt

Directions

- In a large bowl, combine oats, milk, brown sugar, vanilla, cinnamon, and salt. Split between five 8-ounce jars. Toss on the lids and cool overnight or up to 5 days.

Tips

- Tip: People with celiac disease or gluten-sensitivity should use "gluten-free," oats, as oats often become cross-contaminated with wheat and barley.
- To keep it going: Cool for up to 5 days.

Nutrition Info

Serving Size: 2/3 Cup

Per Serving:

197 calories; thiamin 0.2mg ; protein 5.5g; carbohydrates 34.7g ; dietary fiber 4.8g ; magnesium 40.7mg ; folate 19.5mcg ; sugars 7.7g; fat 4.3g ; saturated fat 0.5g ; vitamin a iu 251.9IU ; iron 1.7mg ; vitamin cmg; calcium 251.9mg ; potassium 173.5mg ; sodium 317.8mg ; added sugar 6g.

85. MOZZARELLA PARMESAN STUFFED MUSHROOMS

PREP TIME: 15 minutes

COOK TIME: 15 minutes

TOTAL TIME: 30 minutes

Ingredients

- 12 ounces fresh mushrooms
- 1/2 cup of finely chopped onion
- olive oil (1 tbsp)
- 1 tbsp fresh parsley, minced
- 1/2 tsp basil, dried
- 1/3 cup of Vermouth
- 1 cup of shredded mozzarella

Instructions

1. Remove mushroom stems; set aside caps. Chop stems grossly.
2. Cook chopped mushroom stalks and onions in oil on medium to low heat for 5 minutes or softly. Parsley, basil, and vermouth. Simmer for 10 minutes, or until wine is absorbed; cool for 5 minutes; remove from the sun.
3. Incorporate cheeses. Place the champagne caps with the cheese mixture in 8 to 8-inch baking. Bake in heated 350 degrees F oven 15 minutes or until filling is hot and cheese is melted.

Nutrition

Serving: 2mushrooms | Calories: 123cal | Carbohydrates: 4g | Protein: 7g | Fat: 7g | Saturated Fat: 3g | Cholesterol: 18mg | Sodium: 184mg | Potassium: 213mg | Sugar: 1g | Vitamin A: 220IU | Vitamin C: 3.1mg | Calcium: 147mg | Iron: 0.5mg

86. GARLIC PARMESAN RISOTTO

PREP: 5 minutes

COOK: 20 minutes

TOTAL: 25 minutes

INGREDIENTS

- 1/2 medium onion diced finely
- Four cloves garlic minced
- 1 Tbs olive oil
- 1 Tbs butter
- 4 cups of vegetable stock
- 1/4 cup of dry white wine
- 1 cup of arborio rice
- 1 cup of freshly grated Parmesan cheese plus extra for serving
- 3 Tbs freshly chopped parsley

INSTRUCTIONS

1. Start by heating and keeping your stock warm.
2. In medium heat, add butter and oil to a big pot (I'm using a risotto wok!).
3. Add the onions and cook, then add the garlic until tender. Cook for 1 more minute.

4. Add the rice and coat (making sure oil gets onto every grain of rice if you can) (making sure oil gets onto every grain of rice if you can)
5. 5. Add the wine and blend until it is consumed.
6. Stir in 1 ladle full of stock until it absorbs.
7. Repeat this until almost the entire stock has been used – it should take around 17-25 minutes.
8. Adding the last stock ladle, add the cherry, only let the stock absorb halfway and add your cheese.
9. Let it soak, but not soupy, until it is smooth and thick.
10. Serve, add additional parmesan if desired.

TIPS & NOTES:

- Use white wine for drinking (avoid "cooking wine" labels like the plague). In fact, you won't like the end product if you don't like the wine you use your cooking!
- Don't worry about accurate measuring when you pour into the stock. It simply has to cover the rice surface.
- Gently smell – quick boiling is not what we are looking for.

Using hot stock!! Hot stock helps to keep the rice content in starch.

TABLE OF CONTENTS

CONCLUSION

Made in United States
Troutdale, OR
11/07/2024

24513535R00077